Innovation and Change in I Education

Volume 19

SCOPE OF THE SERIES

The primary aim of this book series is to provide a platform for exchanging experiences and knowledge about educational innovation and change in professional education and post-secondary education (engineering, law, medicine, management, health sciences, etc.). The series provides an opportunity to publish reviews, issues of general significance to theory development and research in professional education, and critical analysis of professional practice to the enhancement of educational innovation in the professions.

The series promotes publications that deal with pedagogical issues that arise in the context of innovation and change of professional education. It publishes work from leading practitioners in the field, and cutting edge researchers. Each volume is dedicated to a specific theme in professional education, providing a convenient resource of publications dedicated to further development of professional education.

Please contact Astrid Noordermeer at Astrid.Noordermeer@springer.com if you wish to discuss a book proposal.

More information about this series at http://www.springer.com/series/6087

Lorelei Lingard • Christopher Watling

Story, Not Study: 30 Brief Lessons to Inspire Health Researchers as Writers

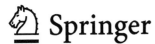 Springer

Lorelei Lingard 🆔
Centre for Education Research
and Innovation
Schulich School of Medicine
& Dentistry
London, ON, Canada

Christopher Watling 🆔
Centre for Education Research
and Innovation
Schulich School of Medicine
& Dentistry
London, ON, Canada

ISSN 1572-1957   ISSN 2542-9957   (electronic)
Innovation and Change in Professional Education
ISBN 978-3-030-71365-2   ISBN 978-3-030-71363-8   (eBook)
https://doi.org/10.1007/978-3-030-71363-8

This Springer imprint is published by the registered company Springer Nature Switzerland AG
The registered company address is: Gewerbestrasse 11, 6330 Cham, Switzerland

We know that writing is hard. It is a stubborn craft, and the process of teasing out a few paragraphs can sometimes be a frustrating one. But there can also be moments of fulfilment – even joy – if we are well-prepared for the task. We hope this book helps you to begin thinking of yourself as a writer, and sets you up to capture a few of those joyful moments.

Foreword

I believe vacations are a sacred time. There are many academics who seem to take pride from working non-stop, often expressed with some form of gleeful (even if not always convincing) claim that they love what they do and, hence, working doesn't really feel like work. I understand the sentiment, but am also of the perspective that the way to maintain that outlook is to give oneself a break when the opportunity arises and something to look forward to in the meantime.

It was in such a state of anticipation that I found myself in late 2020, a year that was built for encouraging vacation if there ever was one. Here, I sat in my makeshift (i.e., socially distanced) home office, blissfully enjoying the dwindling of my pre-holiday to do-list and confident in the belief that everything else could wait until I returned, when I received a request to do more work that I could not refuse.

Before you experience one iota of empathy for my plight, you need to know this tale is the furthest it can be from the classic story of grouchy boss forcing mistreated employee to sit at his desk for long hours in poor conditions. Yes, my home office leaves much to be desired, but sitting in it while being granted the honor of reading and commenting upon a pre-copy of *Story, Not Study* was a welcome gift, not an objectionable chore.

Was I really going to spend part of my far too brief vacation reading a book about writing? You bet your life I was! You see, *Story, Not Study* is not a textbook about writing even though it is rich in practical advice; it is a story unto itself. It's the story of pain and challenge and perseverance that we as academics must all live through. It's a choose-your-own-adventure novel that you, the protagonist, get to decide how to navigate. As a result, how the story resolves is up to you.

I mean that somewhat literally in the sense that Lingard and Watling's clever decision to craft this book as "30 brief lessons" will allow you to read it in almost any order you choose, picking up sections as they become particularly relevant, and returning to them (likely often) for quickly digestible reminders of their sage advice.

I also mean it quite figuratively, however, in the sense that those of us who have chosen health research as a career have a plain choice to make: Either (a) invest the time and energy required to learn how to write well, in the same way we invest to become subject matter experts who have something to write about, or (b) forever be frustrated both by the apparent idiocy of reviewers and editors (particularly editors) who missed something that was *clearly said on page X* and by the suboptimal uptake by readers who *just don't appreciate* the importance of our work.

As an editor and reviewer myself, I'm fully aware that those of us who take on those roles make mistakes. As a scholar in health research, I'm equally aware that our time is limited and that, notions of scientific objectivity be damned, compelling papers are more likely to be read and remembered than less well-written work, even if similar data are on offer. As an author, however, I'm also all too aware that the onus lies upon me to enable readers to understand the message I'm trying to convey rather than blaming them for missing the point.

What is the point in this instance? That writing is bloody hard, that we have no one to fault but ourselves if our message isn't heard, and that avoiding that fate demands the dedicated effort towards skill development that *Story, Not Study* can facilitate. Writing is, after all, a particular skill that deserves to carry all the connotations we apply to other forms of expertise. It requires deliberate practice; it takes time and experience to acquire; it benefits from insightful coaching; it does not allow mindless application of solution algorithms; and, perhaps most importantly, it is not something one can perfect.

To write effectively requires countless decisions and endless trial and error, no matter how long one has been doing it. The choices range from the micro (e.g., how will the tone, meaning, or grammar be impacted by my comma placement?) to the macro (e.g., will this argument be meaningful to the readers I'm trying to reach?) and includes everything in between (e.g., have I structured my paragraphs in a logical way that will allow the key messages to be seen?). Some decisions are a matter of personal style; others are attempts to align with the (current yet unstable) rules of the language or expectations of the genre; others still are matters of with whom one chooses to write and how.

I love, as a result, that Lingard and Watling summarize what they were trying to achieve by offering guidance on this full array of issues by choosing the verb "inspire" (not to mention embedding it right in the title for all to see). In offering their hard-earned lessons, they do much more than teach us how to write well; they demonstrate that it is possible to fall in love with the intellectual puzzles writing presents and encourage us to develop not just the tools, but the motivation to play with words. There is, after all, no one "write" way (pardon the pun) to perform what they have labeled "the craft"; mastering it, to the extent that it can be mastered, requires that we each find our own voice, drawing inspiration, insight, and examples of what works from a wide array of sources, be they other academics, sports columnists, or novelists. There is no better guide to help you along that journey than *Story, Not Study*.

I would advise, as a result, that you not wait until your next holiday to read it.

Editor-in-Chief, Medical Education,   Kevin Eva
Vancouver, Canada

Acknowledgements

We thank the many people who have supported our love of writing and our commitment to creating a writing resource for health researchers. First, we recognize Erik Driessen, Editor of *Perspectives on Medical Education*, for his vision and his faith. Years ago he gave us space in the journal to do something different – The Writer's Craft. A number of the lessons in this book had their first airing in that format, and the refinements here come from thoughtful feedback from writers who took up those lessons and told us what else was needed. Second, we acknowledge our community of researchers and writers at the Centre for Education Research & Innovation, where 'problem-gap-hook' is a verb and candid, enthusiastic discourse about writing is the norm. Third, we thank our Writing Masterclass co-faculty, Sayra Cristancho, Mark Goldszmidt and Kori LaDonna. Our repertoire as writing coaches is enriched by seeing our colleagues adapt, improve and personalize these lessons in their teaching. Finally, we thank the researchers who have trusted us with their writing: graduate students, masterclass participants, junior colleagues and scholarly peers. You've reminded us that there are moments of profound satisfaction to be found amidst the writing struggles we share.

Contents

List of Figures

List of Tables

Chapter 1
Introduction

If you sometimes dread writing, you're not alone. Writing can be tough. Many researchers struggle mightily to put their work into words, only to end up with uninspiring papers that fail to resonate with readers or reviewers. The problem is usually not a lack of effort, but rather a lack of writing training. For many researchers, careful attention to writing is simply not part of their professional preparation. Because they haven't honed the technical skills required to write persuasively, many health researchers rely on intuitive approaches to writing, leaving them with limited versatility. And when writing challenges inevitably present themselves, they lack an inventory of strategies to address them productively.

We aim to change that. This book spotlights the *craft* of scientific writing. Published advice on scientific writing typically shortchanges craft. Instead, it tends toward a checklist-style approach to meeting the minimum bar for publication. We think researchers can reach for a more ambitious goal: a memorable paper that shapes how readers think and feel about a problem that matters.

1.1 Story, Not Study

Our central approach involves a shift in thinking about what we are doing when we write a research paper. Instead of talking about *writing up a study*, we focus on *telling a story*. Great research papers, like great stories, are compelling, memorable, and persuasive. They grab and hold readers' attention, increasing the odds that the research findings will reach and influence their intended audience.

Make no mistake: the notion of *story* here does not imply fiction. Good research stories must be accurate, scientific, and open to critique. Persuasion does not equal deceit. Our storytelling metaphor is not an invitation to gloss over inconvenient results or to make outlandish claims about impact. Rather, it is a framework for crafting papers so that they resonate with their target audience.

© The Author(s), under exclusive license to Springer Nature Switzerland AG 2021
L. Lingard, C. Watling, *Story, Not Study: 30 Brief Lessons to Inspire Health Researchers as Writers*, Innovation and Change in Professional Education 19,
https://doi.org/10.1007/978-3-030-71363-8_1

1

Thinking "Story, Not Study" reinforces several habits that make for great research writing. Stories typically feature "some kind of rupture or disturbance in the normal course of events" (De Fina 2003, p. 13), and bring readers into the actions and reactions that result. A strong research story, likewise, has a "disruption" at its core – a problem that readers will recognize and relate to. Once readers feel the urgency of a problem in their world, their attention will be captured. The story unfolds in the exploration of that problem, and the new insights that exploration yields. Further, stories connect ideas in sensible and meaningful ways. Strong research stories, having captured readers' attention, don't lose them with unproductive detours. Logic and coherence reign. Finally, storytelling "involves persuading an audience that may be skeptical" (Riessman 2008, p. 8). If researchers (and their audiences) lack writing training, they typically do not lack the capacity to critically appraise the research work of others. Strong research writing anticipates the inherent skepticism of its intended audience and doesn't lose sight of their need to be convinced.

As the Pulitzer Prize-winning historian and writer David McCullough noted: "Writing is thinking. To write well is to think clearly. That's why it's so hard" (Cole 2002). Research writing is a difficult business, even for those with considerable experience and training. And that's because writing is unforgiving in revealing the stuff we haven't quite thought through. We can't make connections for our readers until we have made them for ourselves. But we often sit down to write while this all-important thinking process is still incomplete. *Story, Not Study* is thus as much about training thinking as it is training writing. When we craft a research story, we must grapple with how the pieces fit together, and with how that story fits in with conversations in the world we inhabit.

One disclaimer: exceptional writing can't mask shoddy science. There's simply no substitute for research questions that are well-crafted and original, for rigorous methods that align with the study's aims, and for thorough and thoughtful data analysis. The scientific foundation of your work must be solid. Publication efforts can be derailed both by poorly designed and executed studies and by limp, unconvincing scientific storytelling. This guide can only help with the latter!

1.2 Using This Book

The book is divided into three sections – Story, Craft, and Community – each focused on a different element of scientific writing. In the *Story* section, we build the conceptual foundation of a strong paper, introducing concise and coherent strategies to tell research stories. With chapters on each section of a scientific manuscript, from Titles and Abstracts through to Discussions and Limitations, we provide advice on getting the balance of study and story just right. In the *Craft* section, we introduce the grammatical and rhetorical tools of the trade, illustrating how these tools can be wielded for maximum impact. We include chapters on both basic and advanced tools. The former include grammatical fundamentals like constructing high-impact sentences and reining in prepositions and modifiers. The latter delve into more nuanced strategies like gaining mastery of politeness and register in scientific writing. In the *Community* section, we tackle the inherently collaborative nature of contemporary health research writing and highlight its features as a social, rather than a solo, process. The chapters in this section help readers to create and sustain productive writing relationships and communities. Finally, we know that most writers also collaborate with, supervise, and mentor others, and in these roles are called upon to bolster others in their writing endeavors. This section, therefore, also offers a language and a set of strategies for coaching and supporting others.

Each section of the book features an orienting introduction followed by a series of chapters offering short lessons peppered with illustrative examples and handy tables of tips and strategies. The book can be used in its entirety to build holistic writing skills. Graduate students or those newer to research writing might benefit from using the book as a text that helps to ready them for the writing work that lies ahead. But we also encourage the use of chapters as stand-alone lessons – a menu from which to select when targeted skill development is required. Need a grammar refresher? Review the relevant "Basic Tools" chapter. Stuck on the opening paragraph of your Introduction? Review the Problem/Gap/Hook heuristic in Chap. 2. Need to give some difficult writing feedback to a student you're supervising? We've got you covered in Chap. 26.

Our approach is rooted in coaching. We aim to unlock your writerly potential through instruction, reflection, and example. Consistent with this coaching approach, each lesson concludes with an exercise that will prompt you to reflect on your own writing and to experiment with the tools and concepts we have described in order to strengthen that writing. In these exercises, which we have called "See One, Do One, Teach One", we'll ask you to identify dysfunctional patterns in your writing, to try out fixes, and sometimes to use what you have learned to coach others. The exercises aim to create a taste of writing coaching by personalizing the lessons and relating them directly to your own aspirations and goals as a writer. They also aim to support your development of a reflective writing practice, by helping you to recognize, diagnose and improve specific aspects of your writing.

Our book is theoretically informed by writing pedagogy, rhetoric and genre theory, reader cognition research, and linguistic theories of syntax, semantics and pragmatics. However, we've tried to be subtle about it! We've woven this theoretical framing into the chapters, defining important terms and referencing relevant theories, while avoiding extended detours from the practical thrust of the work. We've provided key references at the end of each chapter, however, for those who wish to delve deeper.

1.3 Conclusion

We know that writing is hard. It is a stubborn craft, and the process of teasing out a few paragraphs can sometimes be a frustrating one. But there can also be moments of fulfilment – even joy – if we are well-prepared for the task. We hope this book helps you to begin thinking of yourself as a writer, and sets you up to capture a few of those joyful moments.

References

Cole, B. (2002). A visit with historian David McCullough. *Humanities, 24*(3).
De Fina, A. (2003). *Identity in narrative: A study of immigrant discourse*. Amsterdam: John Benjamins Publishing.
Riessman, C. K. (2008). *Narrative methods for the human sciences*. Thousand Oaks: Sage.

Part I
The Story

When we sit down with our research teams to talk about the manuscript we intend to produce, we typically ask: What's the story? Answering this question activates the *thinking* that underpins sound research writing. Thinking about the story reminds us that we aren't simply documenting findings. We are showing how those findings relate to a problem that means something to our readers. We are convincing them we have an original story to tell – one that builds on, complicates, or challenges the stories others have told. We are persuading them that our research approaches are logical and trustworthy. We are capturing their attention, even when using abbreviated forms of storytelling like titles and abstracts. And we are being honest about the limitations of our work without killing its impact.

In this section, we walk you through each section of a research manuscript, elaborating what needs to be accomplished and highlighting pitfalls that can undermine the work. Of the nine chapters in this section, all but one are relevant regardless of your research paradigm or methodology. The exception is the chapter on presenting your Results. In that chapter, we play to our strengths as qualitative researchers in offering guidance on incorporating quotes in results reporting, but we can't presume to offer meaningful advice on the wide array of other kinds of results that health researchers need to report. Instead, we've followed that oft-repeated advice: write what you know.

Chapter 2
Problem/Gap/Hook Introductions

One of the most powerful shifts a scholarly writer can make has nothing to do with their writing. It has to do with how they think about journals. We tend to think that journals exist to publish scholarly manuscripts. But they don't. They *do* publish scholarly manuscripts, yes, but that is in service of a higher purpose: journals exist to promote scholarly conversations. This chapter orients you to think about your paper as a contribution to a dynamic, even impassioned conversation about a problem in the world that matters.

2.1 Joining a Scholarly Conversation

Kenneth Burke (1974) conceptualized academic writing as an "unending conversation" (pp. 110–111), a heated discussion to which any individual contributor arrives late and from which she departs early. By housing such conversations, journals facilitate a collaborative social process of knowledge building (Thomson and Kamler 2013). And the conversation is becoming increasingly dynamic, as an emerging genre set comprised of invited commentaries, authors' blogs, and podcast author interviews may accompany the publication of original research manuscripts.

Many of us identify as better conversationalists than writers, and the conversation metaphor capitalizes on this strength. Imagine you are not writing a manuscript, but joining a conversation at a social event. After you hang about eavesdropping to get the drift of what's being said (the conversational equivalent of the literature review), you join the conversation with a contribution that signals your shared interest in the topic, your knowledge of what's already been said, and your intention to add something new that will matter to those participating. When you violate any of those expectations, backs turn or eyes roll. Most of us are sufficiently skilled in social etiquette to get this right, at least most of the time. But we don't always apply our social intelligence to scientific communications. We should. Thinking about

© The Author(s), under exclusive license to Springer Nature Switzerland AG 2021
L. Lingard, C. Watling, *Story, Not Study: 30 Brief Lessons to Inspire Health Researchers as Writers*, Innovation and Change in Professional Education 19,
https://doi.org/10.1007/978-3-030-71363-8_2

contributing to a conversation rather than publishing a paper can help to avoid the most common reason for desk rejection: the editor's judgment that "the paper is not relevant for our journal's readership", which translates to "we're not talking about this here".

2.2 The Problem/Gap/Hook Heuristic

The conversation metaphor changes our customary notion of what the Introduction of a scholarly paper is meant to accomplish. To position your work as a compelling conversational turn, your Introduction must do three things: 1. Identify a problem in the world that people are talking about, 2. Establish a gap in the current knowledge or thinking about the problem, and 3. Articulate a hook that convinces readers that this gap is of consequence. Ideally, these three elements appear in the first paragraph or two. Consider this example:

> Providers struggle to navigate communication related to dying and death for patients with chronic illness such as heart failure (HF).[1] Recent discussions articulate communication barriers that must be overcome to systematize and improve decision at the end of life (EOL).[1,2] But HF patients, caregivers, and health care providers (HCPs) remain largely reluctant to communicate about disease progression, prognosis, expectations for future care, death and dying, and palliative care (PC).[3–5] With a growing population of patients facing life-altering health care choices in the context of chronic fatal illnesses like HF, we need to better understand the continuing elusiveness of meaningful and productive discussions for care at the EOL.[6] (Schulz et al. 2017)

In this example, the problem is that providers continue to struggle to communicative effectively about EOL with patients suffering from chronic illness. The gap is that, although knowledge of communication barriers has been used to inform models for systematizing and improving EOL communication, we don't understand why providers are reluctant to implement these models. The hook is that, because the number of patients with chronic fatal illnesses is on the rise, meaningful and effective EOL communication will be increasingly important.

The Problem/Gap/Hook heuristic is relevant regardless of the methodology or domain of your health research manuscript. However, you need to consider how the heuristic might need to be adapted to reflect the conventions in a particularly scholarly conversation. The previous example was from a qualitative research study published in a clinical journal. The next example is the opening paragraph from a survey-based surgical research paper:

> Controversial since its first description in 2012, the ALPPS procedure has demonstrated impressive accelerated liver hypertrophy and expansion of resectability for high liver tumour load, as well as unacceptably high morbidity and mortality.[1, 2, 3, 4, 5, 6, 7, 8, 9, 10, 11, 12, 13] Inconsistent results plague the procedure: some centers report high mortality rates[5, 8] while others report no mortality.[3, 4, 7, 13] The source of this inconsistency is uncertain. Our group hypothesized that variation with respect to indications for surgery, pre-operative decision-making, perioperative care, and surgical technique may explain some of these inconsistencies in published outcomes. This information might be a first step in achieving an

acceptable multicenter morbidity and mortality through international standardization of patient selection, indications and surgical technique. (Buac et al. 2016)

In this example, the problem is that inconsistent results plague a promising surgical procedure, ALPPS. The gap is uncertainty about the source of this inconsistency, and the hook is that, if we understood better why inconsistencies in outcomes exist, we could improve international standardization and identify an acceptable morbidity and mortality to which all centers could aspire. Adapting the Problem/Gap/Hook heuristic to this high impact surgical journal required attention to its convention of presenting the study hypothesis in the first paragraph of the introduction. In stating the hypothesis between the gap and the hook sentences, this paragraph fulfills the convention without sacrificing a compelling and clear introduction.

2.3   Setting Aside the Inverted-Triangle Introduction

In both of the previous examples, the gap statement is preceded by a few sentences of high-level literature review. This 'nod to the known' is a necessary part of the P/G/H formula: making a gap claim without it might suggest to readers that the writer is unaware of the ongoing conversation about the problem. Even with its nod to the known, however, the P/G/H is fundamentally different from the traditional, 'inverted-triangle' introduction. The latter begins broadly and proceeds through a series of literature review paragraphs that gradually narrow onto the focused problem that the manuscript considers. Most scientific writers will have internalized this structure from their high school writing instruction, and it continues to make regular appearances in writing guides, including those for health researchers (e.g., Cunningham et al. 2013). Consider this advice in a commentary on "The art of scientific writing":

> Your high-school English teacher was right: the ideal introduction forms an inverted pyramid starting broad and progressing to specific details. The first paragraph places the work in the broadest possible context.... The second paragraph describes the specific topic addressed in your paper.... The third paragraph describes exactly what was done in your paper. (Plaxo 2010)

Such writing instruction is problematic because it promotes "writing from nowhere" (Crowley 1999) – writing that lacks authentic purpose and specific audience. Student writers in the classroom may feel they have no choice but to adopt the inverted triangle approach to guide a non-differentiated audience from the broadest of disciplinary claims to, finally, the paper's focus. But scientific writers don't need to write from nowhere. Rather, they are joining an ongoing conversation among scholars in their field who care about similar problems and seek to advance knowledge of them. Using broad, general statements as the entrée into an expert and focused conversation is rarely a good strategy. At best it uses up the precious word limit; at worst it tries readers' patience.

It's fine to write your first draft with a broad start, especially if that's how you get your juices flowing. When you revise the piece, however, consider whether you need those broad sentences. Check your introduction for "default" opening lines that may feel redundant to your expert audience. For instance, patient safety researchers will recognize the popular opener:

> Medical error is the leading killer of hospitalized patients in the US, with 44 000 to 98 000 people dying every year.

That is a compelling problem, but it may be too general a lead if the conversation the paper is joining concerns the tensions that arise when health professionals disclose their errors to hospitalized patients and families.

Scientific writers have so effectively internalized the inverted-triangle introduction that they may be reluctant to change. As encouragement, let's consider the advantages of the P/G/H introduction by direct comparison. What follows is an earlier draft of the Buac et al. (2016) introduction written using the inverted triangle approach. In this version, ALPPS did not appear until the second paragraph and the problem of inconsistent results appeared in the third:

> For many patients affected by primary or metastatic hepatic malignancies, liver resection represents the preferential option for cure. A limiting factor for resectability in patients with large tumors or tumors in locations that are difficult to resect is the volume and function of the future liver remnant (FLR). Over the past two decades, various techniques have been employed to induce FLR hypertrophy prior to extensive resections in order to reduce the risk of postoperative liver failure. These techniques manipulate and redistribute portal venous blood flow to the liver by portal vein occlusion of specific branches. This results in FLR hypertrophy that aims to convert unresectable cases to resectable ones. Two-stage hepatectomy is a liver resection performed in two stages. because the tumor burden cannot be removed in one stage. It has been developed for the treatment of bilobar tumours and can be combined with portal vein occlusion to induce hypertrophy between the two stages (ie. portal vein embolization or ligation).[1–7] The most significant causes for failure to complete surgical resection after portal vein occlusion have been reported to be progression of the disease during the interval between the two stages (10%) and insufficient hypertrophy of the FLR (2%).[8]
>
> ALPPS (Associating Liver Partitioning and Portal Vein Ligation for Staged Hepatectomy) has emerged as another technique to resolve this problem. It is a two-stage procedure that combines portal vein ligation and in-situ parenchymal transection of the liver, with the objective to increase resectability rate by extensive and accelerated FLR hypertrophy. This procedure was first performed in 2007 by Dr. Hans Schlitt in Germany and the technique was first reported in 2012.[9] Since that inaugural description, ALPPS has been carried out in many centers worldwide. Several studies have demonstrated impressive hypertrophy with a 60-90% increase in volume between stages 1 and 2, with almost all patients going on to complete the second stage with an R0 resection.[9–21] However, since the first landmark study reported a 12% 90-day mortality[9] and subsequent reports confirmed this high risk,[10,13,14,16] ALPPS has also been plagued by skepticism. This has culminated in calls for caution from experienced liver centers,[22,23] formation of an international registry to assess safety, and controversial discussion at recent hepatobiliary meetings.
>
> ALPPS mortality rates and complications vary widely across centers. While some centers reported mortality rates up to 22% and 29%,[13,16] others have reported no mortalities in their series.[11,12,15,21] ALPPS has also been associated with a high rate of severe complications (Clavien-Dindo classification over IIIB), with some series reporting up to 28%.[14] The first

analysis of the international registry reported that the rate of post-operative liver failure by 50-50 criteria is 9% after either the first or second stage of ALPPS.[14] This report also concluded that indications play a major role in determining outcomes. The use of ALPPS for primary liver tumors was associated with a high morbidity and mortality, especially in elderly patients. The study also demonstrated that a prolonged stage 1 with operating time over 5 hours, as well as the need for blood transfusions, yielded inferior outcomes. Many technical variations on the original ALPPS technique have been developed in an attempt to improve outcomes. This includes the non-touch anterior approach,[24–26] the "hybrid ALPPS" which combines parenchymal transection with portal vein embolization,[27] the use of a liver tourniquet rather than an in-situ split of liver parenchyma,[18] radio-frequency assisted liver partition (RALPP),[28] laparoscopic ALPPS,[29–31] as well as a myriad of modifications regarding which segments of the liver are resected and preserved.[32–34] (Hernandez 2020)

In the revisions towards the published P/G/H version (Buac et al. 2016), the authors of the ALPPS paper decided that, because they were joining a scholarly conversation among liver resection experts, the first paragraph explaining the challenges associated with liver resection was unnecessary. Furthermore, they wanted to bring the problem of inconsistent results into focus sooner than the inverted triangle logic allowed.

When you begin a scientific manuscript with a Problem/Gap/Hook introductory paragraph, the remainder of the introduction must backfill the evidence for the claims asserted up front. In the published Buac et al. (2016) paper, for instance, the second paragraph reviews the evidence for unacceptably high mortality and morbidity with ALPPS, the third paragraph reviews the evidence regarding more promising outcomes, and the fourth summarizes existing theories about the source of this inconsistency. The key is not to simply repeat the Problem/Gap/Hook claims, but to elaborate and evidence them in the following paragraphs.

2.4   Tips for an Effective Problem/Gap/Hook

A few distinctions may be helpful as you conceptualize the Problem/Gap/Hook for your paper. First, the problem you're exploring is not the same as the topic. The following introductory sentence states the topic:

Team communication plays an important role in patient safety.

While this version states a problem:

Adverse events resulting from error happen at unacceptably high rates in hospital, and ineffective communication among team members is often a contributing factor.

Notice the greater sense of urgency – a problem in the world that matters – conveyed by the second example.

Second, the Problem/Gap/Hook is not the same as your research question and purpose statement. While a clear question and purpose are undoubtedly important features of a research study, they are not the most powerful entrée into a scholarly conversation. Consider these two examples. The first centers on the question and purpose, while the second uses a Problem/Gap/Hook structure.

> Leadership is increasingly recognized as an important competency for physicians. At the same time, collaboration is growing as a value and expectation of healthcare delivery. What has not been explored is the relationship between leadership and collaboration in physicians' practice. The purpose of this study was to explore this relationship by asking "How do physicians experience leadership and collaboration during their daily team interactions?"

> Leadership and collaboration are highly valued but potentially conflicting competencies in medical practice. While there has been attention to leadership and to collaboration individually, little attention has been paid to how they interact. With physicians experiencing increasingly formal expectations that they will lead and collaborate effectively, (e.g., CanMEDS 2015), we require systematic knowledge about how these competencies play out in clinical teams.

Both introductions summarize a gap in knowledge effectively. But the second one, by opening with a problem – these are 'highly valued but potentially conflicting competencies' – grabs the reader's attention and inserts itself forcefully into conversations about leadership, collaboration, and competency-based education.

Third, thinking critically about your Problem, Gap and Hook can help you to identify aspects of your Introduction where you may be need to be strategic. For instance, are you writing about a novel problem for which there is currently no ongoing scholarly conversation? This is a rare event and, if you think it applies to you, check the literature again. But it does happen: an example might be the first cost analysis following the implementation of medical assistance in dying in Canada. Are you writing about a problem that is currently being explored, such as how to increase organ donation rates? Or are you writing about a problem that some readers might see as passé or already solved, such as how to implement interprofessional education activities across undergraduate health sciences programs? Each of these situations requires a slightly different strategy. Is the gap you have identified one that readers are likely to agree upon, or is there debate about whether more knowledge is required in this area? If readers do not believe that the gap *exists*, then they may assume your literature review is flawed. If they do not agree that the gap *matters* – that is, that filling it will change anything – then your story will have no 'hook' to draw them in.

Finally, when crafting your hook, try it more than one way. A positive hook expresses the 'so what' in terms of possibilities, using language such as "With this knowledge, we can better address..." or "This work offers a critical step towards...". A negative hook expresses the 'so what' in terms of cautions, with language such as "Without systematic exploration, we risk..." or "Until we understand this phenomenon, we cannot...". Neither kind of hook is right or wrong *per se*; it's a matter of best fit with the problem as you've outlined it.

2.5 Conclusion

The Problem/Gap/Hook heuristic can help focus both your writing and your thinking. Try using it as you brainstorm a thesis project with students or sketch a grant
application with collaborators. Articulating the P/G/H early and iterating it often is a
way of ensuring that your team has clarity about the problem you'll tackle, certainty
about the gap you'll fill, and confidence about why filling the gap is worth your
efforts, funders' support, and readers' attention.

The Problem/Gap/Hook heuristic is most useful if you remember that research
dissemination is a social and rhetorical act. Journals are static artifacts, but the
conversations that they support are dynamic. The Problem/Gap/Hook heuristic is a
powerful way to shape your introduction so that it participates in this scholarly
conversation.

See One, Do One, Teach One
Complete the following four sentences to draft a P/G/H paragraph

(Problem) The problem is...
(Nod to the Known) What we know is...
(Gap) What we don't know is...
(Hook) And this matters because...

Partner with a colleague from your writing community and tell each other your
P/G/H paragraphs orally. Give each other feedback using the language of the
heuristic. For example:

- "I think I heard two problems instead of just one. Did you intend that?"
- "The nod to the known is pretty elaborate. It might be overshadowing the
  gap. Is some of it more critical than the rest?"
- "The gap was clear to me: this is what I understood . . ."
- "I didn't hear a hook."
- "I heard a negative hook but it felt a bit overstated to me. Does it really limit
  future patient care if you don't fill the gap you've identified?"

References

Buac, S., Schadde, E., Schnitzbauer, A. A., Vogt, K., & Hernandez-Alejandro, R. (2016). The many
   faces of ALPPS: Surgical indications and techniques among surgeons collaborating in the
   international registry. *HPB, 18*(5), 442–448. https://doi.org/10.1016/j.hpb.2016.01.547.
Burke, K. (1974). *The philosophy of literary form: Studies in symbolic action* (3rd ed.). Berkeley:
   University of California Press.
Crowley, S. (1999). The universal requirement in first-year composition. *Basic Writing e-Journal, 1*
   (2). https://bwe.ccny.cuny.edu/Issue%201.2.html#sharon.
Cunningham, C. J. L., Weathington, B. L., & Pittenger, D. J. (2013). *Understanding and
   conducting research in the health sciences*. Hoboken: Wiley.
Hernandez-Alejandro, R. (2020). *Permission to reproduce draft*. Personal email communication.

Plaxco, K. W. (2010). The art of writing science. *Protein Science, 19*(12), 2261–2266. https://doi. org/10.1002/pro.514.

Schulz, V., Crombeen, A., Marshall, D., Shadd, J., LaDonna, K., & Lingard, L. (2017). Beyond simple planning: Existential dimensions of conversations with patients at risk of dying from heart failure. *Journal of Pain and Symptom Management, 54*(5), 637–644. https://doi.org/10. 1016/j.jpainsymman.2017.07.041.

Thomson, P., & Kamler, B. (2013). *Writing for peer-reviewed journals: Strategies for getting published*. London: Routledge.

Chapter 3
Mapping the Gap

This chapter and the next offer strategies for effectively presenting the literature review section of a research manuscript. In this chapter, we alert writers to the importance of not only summarizing what is known but also identifying precisely what is not, in order to explicitly signal the relevance of their research. We introduce readers to the "mapping the gap" metaphor, the knowledge claims heuristic, and the need to characterize the gap.

3.1 Mapping the Gap

The purpose of the literature review section of a manuscript is not to report what is known about your topic. The purpose is to identify what remains *unknown* – what academic writing scholars have called the "knowledge deficit" (Giltrow et al. 2014) – thus establishing the need for your research study. In the previous chapter, the Problem/Gap/Hook heuristic was introduced as a way of opening your paper with a clear statement of the problem that your work grapples with, the gap in our current knowledge about that problem, and the reason the gap matters. This chapter explains how to use the literature review section of your paper to build and characterize the gap claim in your Problem/Gap/Hook. The metaphor of "mapping the gap" is a way of thinking about how to select and arrange your review of the existing literature so that readers can recognize why your research needed to be done, and why its results constitute a meaningful advance on what was already known.

Many writers have learned that the literature review should describe what is known. The trouble with this approach is that it can produce a laundry list of 'facts-in-the-world' that does not persuade the reader that the current study is a necessary next step. Instead, think of your literature review as painting in a map of your research domain: as you review existing knowledge, you are painting in

L. Lingard, C. Watling, *Story, Not Study: 30 Brief Lessons to Inspire Health Researchers as Writers*, Innovation and Change in Professional Education 19, https://doi.org/10.1007/978-3-030-71363-8_3

sections of the map, but your goal is not to end with the whole map fully painted. That would mean there is nothing more we need to know about the topic, and that leaves no room for your research. What you want to end up with is a map in which painted sections surround and emphasize a white space, a gap in what is known that matters. Conceptualizing your literature review this way helps to ensure that it achieves its dual goal of presenting what is known and pointing out what is not. The latter of these goals is necessary for your literature review to establish the necessity and importance of the research you will describe in the methods section.

To a novice researcher or graduate student, this may seem counterintuitive. Hopefully you have invested significant time in reading the existing literature, and you are understandably keen to demonstrate that you've read everything ever published about your topic! Be careful, though, not to use the literature review section to regurgitate all of your reading in manuscript form. For one thing, it creates a laundry list of facts that makes for horrible reading. But there are three other reasons for avoiding this approach. First, you don't have the space. In published health research papers, the literature review is customarily quite short, ranging from a few paragraphs to a few pages, so you can't summarize everything you've read. Second, you're preaching to the converted. If you approach your paper as a contribution to an ongoing scholarly conversation, then your literature review should summarize just the aspects of that conversation that are required to situate *your* conversational turn as informed and relevant. Third, the key to relevance is to point to *a gap* in what is known. To do so, you summarize what is known for the express purpose of *identifying what is not known*. Seen this way, the literature review should exert a gravitational pull on the reader, leading them inexorably to the white space on the map of knowledge you've painted for them. That white space is the space that your research fills.

The gap is not something that readers should have to infer: it should be explicitly stated and proven as part of the literature review. Not uncommonly though, the literature review sections of published papers end with a statement like this:

> A better understanding of underlying stressors and coping mechanisms is needed to address the increasing rates of burnout within [this specialty].

This statement implies a gap, but it neither states nor evidences one. Consider this revision, which summarizes the key knowledge claims from the literature review as way of spotlighting the gap:

> Given the strong evidence placing [this specialty] at high risk of burnout and the increasing national shortage of [these specialists] promising to exacerbate this situation, the lack of research into underlying stressors and coping mechanisms in [this specialty] presents a critical barrier to resolving this situation.

The phrase "lack of research" explicitly signals the gap, which is further emphasized as being "a critical barrier" to moving the scholarly conversation forward.

3.2 Knowledge Claims

To help writers move beyond the laundry list of facts, the notion of 'knowledge claims' can be useful. A knowledge claim is a way of presenting the growing understanding of the community of researchers who have been exploring your topic. These are not disembodied facts, but rather incremental insights that some in the field may agree with and some may not, depending on their different methodological and disciplinary approaches to the topic. Treating the literature review as a story of the knowledge claims being made by researchers in the field can help writers with one of the most sophisticated aspects of a literature review – locating the knowledge being reviewed. Where does it come from? What are its limits? Under what conditions and from which positions does it arise? How do different methodologies influence the knowledge being accumulated? And so on.

Consider this example of the knowledge claims (KC), gap and hook for the literature review section of a research paper on distributed healthcare teamwork:

KC	We know that poor team communication can cause errors.
KC	And we know that team training can be effective in improving team communication.
KC	This knowledge has prompted a push to incorporate teamwork training principles into health professions education curricula.
KC	However, most of what we know about team training research has come from research with co-located teams – i.e., teams whose members work together in time and space.
Gap	Little is known about how teamwork training principles would apply in distributed teams, whose members work asynchronously and are spread across different locations.
Hook	Given that much healthcare teamwork is distributed rather than co-located, our curricula will be severely lacking until we create refined teamwork training principles that reflect distributed as well as co-located work contexts.

The 'We know that…' structure illustrated in this example is a template for helping you draft and organize. In your final version, your knowledge claims will be expressed with more sophistication. For instance, "We know that poor team communication can cause errors" will become something like "Over a decade of patient safety research has demonstrated that poor team communication is the dominant cause of medical errors." This simple template of knowledge claims, though, provides an outline for the paragraphs in your literature review, each of which will provide detailed evidence to illustrate a knowledge claim. Using this approach, the order of the paragraphs in the literature review is strategic and persuasive, leading the reader to the gap claim that positions the relevance of the current study.

As you organize your knowledge claims, you will also want to consider whether you are trying to map the gap in a relatively understudied field or well-studied one. The rhetorical challenge is different in each case. In an understudied field, the challenge is not proving that a gap exists, it is proving that the gap matters. There are many unknowns in any health research field: some clearly matter to current conversations and others may appear more tangential. Your literature review must map a new gap in a way that establishes it as a priority and as relevant to pressing concerns. By contrast, in a well-studied field such as professionalism in medical education, you must make a strong, explicit case for the *existence* of a gap. Readers may come to your paper tired of hearing about this topic and tempted to think that we can't possibly need more knowledge about it. Listing the knowledge claims can help you organize them most effectively and determine which pieces of knowledge may be unnecessary to map the white space your research attempts to fill. This does not mean that you leave out relevant information: your literature review must still be accurate. But, since you will not be able to include everything, selecting carefully among the possible knowledge claims is essential to producing a coherent, well-argued literature review.

3.3   Characterizing the Gap

Once you've identified the gap, your literature review must characterize it. What *kind* of gap have you found? There are many ways to characterize a gap, but some of the more common are a pure knowledge deficit, a shortcoming (usually conceptual or methodological) in the scholarship, a controversy, and a pervasive, unproven assumption. Table 3.1 illustrates each of these:

Pure knowledge gaps are rare, and the suspicion that you've found one should send every writer back to the literature to double check. The next two kinds of knowledge gap are not necessarily mutually exclusive, and it can be a matter of

Table 3.1 Characterizing the gap

Type of gap	A deficit	A shortcoming	A controversy	An assumption
Example	No known research has looked at the experience of medical student abuse within longitudinal integrated clerkships.	Much research has surveyed the frequency of medical errors committed by residents. However, these survey results have not offered insight into residents' subjective experience of their errors.	Scholars disagree on the impact of fatigue on the quality of medical care.	The theme of technological heroism – technology will solve what ails us – is ubiquitous in the literature on health systems reform, but what is that belief based on?

rhetorical positioning whether the writer characterizes the gap more as a shortcoming or as a controversy. Take the following published example:

> Despite such clear uptake of and enthusiasm in the CW [Choosing Wisely] initiative and some early successes in lowering low-value care through local interventions,[10–14] studies have shown limited large-scale change in ordering rates of low-value care since the launch of these campaigns.[15,16] The issue of implementing CW recommendations and evaluating the effects of these recommendations has received much less attention. Recommendations alone will not change practice.[17,18] Recent commentaries have suggested that the focus of the campaign should be on identifying and applying evidence-based strategies to effectively reduce low-value care.[13–19] There is substantial evidence and guidance on how to implement evidence-based strategies. However, few conceptual frameworks exist to guide de-implementation, and those that do exist focus on team culture or organisational change[20] or target change in a specific clinical setting,[21] making it difficult to generalise the frameworks across a myriad of healthcare settings and contexts. (Grimshaw et al. 2020)

The paragraph's first sentence offers a sense of controversy by using "Despite" and setting up a sharp contrast between "clear uptake of and enthusiasm in CW" and "limited large-scale change". The second sentence identifies a shortcoming: "much less attention" has been paid to implementation and evaluation. The sense of a controversy in the scholarly conversation around CW returns in the third, strongly worded sentence: "Recommendations alone will not change practice." The reader has a sense of camps in the CW debate, and of the writers' attempt to turn the discussion away from recommendations and towards the nuances of de-implementation. The last sentence returns to characterizing the gap as a shortcoming in scholarship, asserting that "few conceptual frameworks exist to guide de-implementation, and those that do exist focus on team culture or organisational change or target change in a specific clinical setting" (Grimshaw et al. 2020, p. 410). These writers effectively characterize the space their work fills as both a controversy and a shortcoming – these two kinds of gap can be complementary. Deciding how to characterize the gap when it has the potential to be defined in multiple ways is part of the art of storytelling in a manuscript. The authors of the previous example could arguably have presented the gap as merely a shortcoming and not also a controversy. The story, however, would not have been as compelling.

To characterize the kind of gap, you need to know the literature thoroughly. That means more than understanding each paper individually; you also need to be placing each paper in relation to others, and understanding how, together, they map what Giltrow et al. (2014) refer to as the 'state of knowledge.' This may require changing your note-taking technique while you're reading; take notes on what each paper contributes to knowledge, but also on how it relates to other papers you've read, and what it suggests about the kind of gap that is emerging.

3.4 Conclusion

In summary, think of your literature review as mapping the gap rather than simply summarizing the known. And pay attention to characterizing the kind of gap you've mapped. This strategy can help to make your literature review into a compelling argument rather than a list of facts. It can remind you of the danger of describing so fully what is known that the reader is left with the sense that there is no pressing need to know more. And it can help you to establish a coherence between the kind of gap you've identified and the study methodology you will use to fill it.

> **See One, Do One, Teach One**
> Using the template below, create a knowledge claims table for your story. You may wish to begin with the gap you propose to fill. Phrases for starting the gap sentence are suggested. Now, working backwards, write three knowledge claims that map the space around this gap in the literature. Use "we know that" to start each sentence: you can finesse the language in a later revision. Support each knowledge claim with at least one reference.
>
> | Knowledge Claim | We know that … | References |
> |---|---|---|
> | Knowledge Claim | We know that … | |
> | Knowledge Claim | We know that … | |
> | GAP | However…
 But…
 Notwithstanding these advances… | |
>
> Speak the knowledge claims and gap claim aloud: are there any implicit jumps in logic that need to be filled? If so, add knowledge claims until the logic is explicit and sound, and the sentences draw the reader convincingly to the gap your work fills.

References

Giltrow, J., Gooding, R., Burgoyne, D., & Sawatsky, M. (2014). *Academic writing: An introduction* (3rd ed.). Peterborough: Broadview Press.

Grimshaw, J. M., Patey, A. M., Kirkham, K. R., Hall, A., Dowling, S. K., Rodondi, N., et al. (2020). De-implementing wisely: Developing the evidence base to reduce low-value care. *BMJ Quality & Safety, 29*(5), 409–417. https://doi.org/10.1136/bmjqs-2019-010060.

Chapter 4
Citation Technique

This chapter continues our consideration of strategies for effectively presenting the literature review section of a research manuscript. Here we argue that citation is not just a technical practice but also a rhetorical one, and we offer writers an expanded vocabulary for using citation to maximal effect.

4.1 Citation Strategies

Many writers think of citation as the formal system we use to avoid plagiarism and acknowledge others' work. But citation is a much more nuanced practice than this. Not only does citation allow us to represent the source of knowledge, but also it allows us to position ourselves in relation to that knowledge, and to place that knowledge in relation to other knowledge. In short, citation is how we artfully tell the story of what the field knows, how it came to that knowledge, and where we stand in relation to it as we write the literature review section to frame our own work. Seen this way, citation is a sophisticated task, requiring in-depth knowledge of the literature in a domain.

Citation is more than just referencing; it is how we represent the social construction of knowledge in a field. A citation strategy is any indication in the text about the source and nature of knowledge. Consider the following passage, in which all citation strategies are bolded:

Despite years of effort to teach and enforce positive professional norms and standards, **many reports of** challenges to medical professionalism **continue to appear, both in the medical and education literature and, often in reaction, in the lay press.**[1,2,3,4,5] Examples of professional lapses dot the health care landscape: regulations are thwarted, records are falsified, patients are ignored, colleagues are berated.[2,4,6] **The medical profession has articulated its sense** of what professionalism is **in a number of important position statements.**[7,8] **These statements** tend to be **built upon** abstracted principles and values, such as the taxonomy **presented in the American Board of Internal Medicine's (ABIM's)**

© The Author(s), under exclusive license to Springer Nature Switzerland AG 2021
L. Lingard, C. Watling, *Story, Not Study: 30 Brief Lessons to Inspire Health Researchers as Writers*, Innovation and Change in Professional Education 19,
https://doi.org/10.1007/978-3-030-71363-8_4

Project Professionalism: altruism, accountability, excellence, duty, honor, integrity, and respect for others.[7] (Ginsburg et al. 2002, p. 516)

In this passage, citation as referencing (in the form of Vancouver format super-script numbers) is used to acknowledge the source of knowledge. There are more than just references in this passage, however. Citation strategies also include statements that characterize the density of that knowledge ("many reports"), its temporal patterns ("continue to appear"), its diverse origins ("both in the medical and education literature"), its social nature ("often in reaction"), and its social import ("important position statements"). As you can see, citation does more than just acknowledge the source of something you've read. It is how you represent the social nature of knowledge as coming from somewhere, being debated and developed, and having impact on the world (Giltrow et al. 2014). If we remove all these citation strategies, the passage from Ginsburg et al. sounds at best like common sense or, at worst, like unsubstantiated personal opinion:

> Despite years of effort to teach and enforce positive professional norms and standards, challenges to medical professionalism continue. Examples of professional lapses dot the health care landscape: regulations are thwarted, records are falsified, patients are ignored, colleagues are berated. Professionalism is a set of principles and values: altruism, account-ability, excellence, duty, honor, integrity, and respect for others.

4.2   Taking a Stance

Perhaps you have been told that your literature review should be 'objective' – that you should simply present what is known without taking a stance on it. This is largely untrue, for two reasons. The first involves the distinction between summary and critical summary. A summary is a neutral description of material, but a good literature review contains very little pure summary because, as we review, we must also judge the quality, source and reliability of the knowledge claims we're presenting. To do this, we engage in *critical* summary, not only summarizing existing knowledge but offering a stance on it.

The second reason is that, even when we're aiming for simple summary, a completely neutral presentation of knowledge claims is very difficult to achieve. We take a stance in ways we hardly even notice. Consider how the verb in each of these statements adds a flavor of stance to what is otherwise a summary of a knowledge claim in the field:

> Anderson describes how the assessment is overly time-consuming for use in the Emergency Department.
>   Anderson discovered that the assessment was overly time-consuming for use in the Emergency Department.
>   Anderson claims that the assessment is overly time-consuming for use in the Emergency Department.

The first verb, 'describes', is neutral: it is not possible to ascertain the writer's stance on the knowledge Anderson has contributed to the field. The second verb,

Table 4.1 Verbs to position the writer in relation to the literature being reviewed

Neutral about the knowledge		Affiliating with the knowledge		Distancing from the knowledge	
Comments	observes	discovers	addresses	assumes	hopes
explains	remarks	reveals	argues	claims	believes
indicates	states	realizes	recognizes	contends	*suggests*
notes	finds	understands	identifies	argues	
describes	*suggests*	clarifies	demonstrates		

Table 4.2 Verbs to represent the nature and strength of an author's contributions to the literature

Verbs to report what an author DID	Verbs to report what an author SAID		Verbs to report an author's OPINION	
analyse, assess, <u>conclude</u>, discover, describe, demonstrate, examine, explore, establish, find, identify, inquire, prove, observe, study, show	Weaker	Stronger	Weaker	Stronger
	comment	affirm	accept	argue
	describe	emphasize	believe	assert
	note	stress	consider	claim
	remark	maintain	think	contend
	add	stipulate	<u>suggest</u>	deny
	offer	explain	suspect	recommend
	<u>suggest</u>	<u>conclude</u>	speculate	reject
		identify		advocate
		insist		maintain

'discovered', expresses an affiliation or positive stance in the writer, while the third verb, 'claims', distances the writer from Anderson's work. Even these brief summary sentences contain a flavor of critical summary. This is not a flaw: in fact, it is an important method of portraying existing knowledge as a conversation in which the writer is positioning themselves and their work. But it should be done consciously and strategically. Table 4.1 offers examples to help writers think about how the verbs in their literature review position them in relation to existing knowledge in the field. Meaning is subject to context and these examples should only be taken as a guide: e.g., "suggests" can be used to signal neutrality or distancing.

Most of us have favorite verbs that we default to almost unconsciously when we're writing – reports, argues, describes, studies, explains, asserts – but these verbs are not interchangeable. They each inscribe a slightly different stance towards the knowledge – not only the writer's stance, but also the stance of the researcher who created the knowledge. It is critical to get the original stance right in your critical summary. Nothing irritates an author more than seeing her stance misrepresented in someone else's literature review. For example, if Lorelei wrote a paragraph offering tentative reflections on a new idea, she doesn't want to see that summarized in someone's literature review as "Lingard argues", when more accurate would be "Lingard suggests" or "Lingard explored".

Writers need to extend their library of citation verbs to allow themselves to accurately and persuasively position knowledge claims published by authors in their field. You can find many online resources to help extend your vocabulary; Table 4.2, adapted from one such online source (University of Portsmouth 2017), provides some suggestions. Tables like these should be thought of as tools, not rules.

Table 4.3   Verbs to express relations among authors in the field

Depicting similar positions	Depicting contrasting positions	Depicting relating/responding positions
Taylor acknowledges Jackson's claim that... affirms, agrees, confirms, concurs, aligns, shares, echoes, supports, verifies, concedes, accepts	Taylor refutes Jackson's claim that... argues, disagrees, questions, dismisses, refuses, rejects, challenges, contradicts, criticizes, opposes, counters, disputes	Taylor adds to Jackson's claim that... extends, elaborates, refines, builds on, reconsiders, draws upon, advances, repositions, addresses

Keep in mind that words have flexible meanings depending on context and purpose. This is why one word, such as suggest or conclude, can appear in more than one list.

Knowledge is a social construction and it accumulates as researchers debate, extend and refine one another's contributions. To avoid your literature review reading like a laundry list of disconnected facts, reporting verbs are an important resource. Table 4.3 offers a selection of verbs organized to reflect different relationships among authors in the field of knowledge being reviewed.

Finally, although we have focused on citation verbs in this chapter, adverbs (e.g., similarly, consequently) and prepositional phrases (e.g., by contrast, in addition) are also important for expressing similar, contrasting or responding relations among knowledge claims and their authors in the field being reviewed. See Chaps. 15 and 16.

Critical summary requires writers to take a stance. That can be difficult, as stance is rooted in implicit values – in a way of approaching the world that becomes habituated until it seems like no stance at all. Precise writers must not allow their own stance to become unconscious. Instead, they should treat stance as an explicit technique that requires self-reflection, asking "what is my stance in relation to this knowledge, why is it so, has it changed, and, if so, why and how"? This is true whether we are longstanding participants in a scholarly conversation who may wish to alter our prior stance, or relative newcomers to the conversation who may wish to hedge cautiously amidst heated debate. In either case, Graff and Birkenstein's (2018) templates for primary critical stances can provide useful tools for making stance conscious while drafting the literature review, and for stepping back and assessing it as you revise and refine. Figure 4.1 draws on Graff and Birkenstein's template approach to sketch three primary stances: agreeing, with a difference; disagreeing, with reasons; and agreeing and disagreeing simultaneously.

4.3   Conclusion

In summary, an effective literature review not only summarizes existing knowledge, it also critically presents that knowledge to depict an evolving conversation in a particular domain of study. As writers we need to know when we are summarizing

---

Agreeing, with a difference:

X's argument that _____ also applies to the problem of _____.
The theory of _____ holds in this situation because _____.

Disagreeing, with reasons:

By emphasizing _____, X overlooks the larger question of _____.
X's argument for _____ depends on the problematic assumption that _____.

Agreeing & disagreeing simultaneously

While _____ resonates with recent research, it fails to explain how _____.
Although I recognize the value of _____, I remain unconvinced that _____.

Fig. 4.1 Three approaches to stance

and when we are critically summarizing – summary alone makes for a literature review that reads like a list of undigested 'facts-in-the-world'. Finally, writers need to attend to the subtle power of citation terms such as verbs, adverbs and prepositions to position themselves and the authors they are citing in relation to the knowledge being reviewed. Broadening our catalogue of 'go-to' verbs, in particular, can enliven and strengthen our writing.

See One, Do One, Teach One
1. If your literature review feels without stance, ask someone else to read it and flag when they see you using one of the three primary stances in Fig. 4.1.
2. Circle all the reporting verbs in your literature. What are your default verbs? Using Tables 4.1, 4.2 and 4.3 as a resource, revise your verbs to express your own position on the knowledge and to represent relations among scholars in the field.
3. Identify a key source you plan to cite in your literature review, and practice taking a stance. Experiment with expressing agreement and affiliation or disagreement and distance. Notice how stance shifts as you modify your verb choices.

References

Giltrow, J., Gooding, R., Burgoyne, D., & Sawatsky, M. (2014). *Academic writing: An introduction* (3rd ed.). Peterborough: Broadview Press.
Ginsburg, S., Regehr, G., Stern, D., & Lingard, L. (2002). The anatomy of the professional lapse: Bridging the gap between traditional frameworks and students' perceptions. *Academic Medicine, 77*(6), 516–522. https://doi.org/10.1097/00001888-200206000-00007.

Graff, G., & Birkenstein, C. (2018). *"They say/I say": The moves that matter in academic writing* (4th ed.). New York: W.W Norton.

University of Portsmouth. (2017).*Writing about others' work: Verbs for citations.* Department of Curriculum and Quality Enhancement. https://www.port.ac.uk/student-life/help-and-advice/study-skills/research-reading-referencing-and-citation/verbs-for-citations. Accessed 8 Sept 2020.

Chapter 5
Methods: Where Story Meets Study

Our "story not study" mantra seeks to inspire writers of scientific manuscripts to aim for papers that are at once accurate and artful. But if any element of a research paper can feel an uneasy fit with this ethos, it is the Methods section. Here, we bring the study to the fore, exposing its foundations and blueprints. Laden with logistics, the Methods section can seem instrumental. Indeed, most of the published guidance on writing this section focuses entirely on content – the *stuff* that needs to populate that section of your paper – rather than on craft. But there is an art to writing methods well. Clarity and persuasion are as critical here as elsewhere in your paper. Writing your methods in a way that advances and aligns with your research story demands attention not only to what you include, but also to what you need to accomplish. Good Methods writing demands that we commit, justify, explain, educate, anticipate, and reflect. Let's consider each of these elements.

5.1 Commit

Commit to a methodology and name it whenever possible. This one sounds simple, but it is easy to overlook. If you have done a constructivist grounded theory study, say so. If you have opted for a randomized controlled trial, tell us that. While methods are the tools of the trade, *methodology* is the philosophy that guides how and when you deploy those tools. Ideally, then, open your Methods section with an explicit nod to a specific methodology. Doing so is like letting readers know what language you will be speaking; it helps them to know what to expect, alerts them to your design orientation, and enables them to judge the quality of the work. And if you have blended methodologies or departed significantly from your chosen methodological path, then you must explicitly work to help readers overcome their potential sense of disorientation or incoherence. Don't wait till the Limitations: you will have lost them already.

5.2   Justify

Most research questions can be approached in more than one way. Your goal, therefore, is to present the approach you selected as the *obvious* choice (Kotz and Cals 2013). A reviewer's lingering sense that the study would have been more effectively done using an entirely different set of methods can be fatal; the last thing you want to read in a review is a line that begins "I wish that the authors had instead chosen...".

Justifying your methodological choices can mitigate such critiques and reassure readers that your approach – whether it is familiar to them or not – is fundamentally sound. Justification may need to be woven strategically through the Methods section. Tell readers why the methodology you have selected is the right match for your research question. Describe the particular affordances of your research setting and context for the questions at hand. Offer reasons for your sampling strategy. If sampling purposively, for example, tell readers why you anticipated that the particular participants you recruited would be usefully informative. For example, instead of stopping at "We recruited 20 surgical residents for this study of how teacher-learner relationships influence feedback practices", offer a rationale for that sampling choice:

> We recruited 20 surgical residents for this study of how teacher-learner relationships influence feedback practices. We chose to study surgical residents because surgical training typically involves teacher-learner pairs who spend extended periods of time working together in the operating room. We therefore anticipated that surgical residents might be especially well-positioned to offer insights into our research questions.

Justifying key design decisions reassures readers and reviewers that the approach is well considered and robust.

Pragmatic decisions often need to be made in the course of a research project. Sometimes the original approach to recruiting participants doesn't pay the anticipated dividends, and a "plan B" is required. Or perhaps unforeseen circumstances mean that faculty training that was intended to be done in-person needs to be delivered remotely. Research, particularly when it is conducted in real clinical settings, involves a lot of moving parts, and researchers sometimes need to be adaptable. But when you adapt your plan, you need to offer a convincing rationale for the choices you made, so that you maintain your readers' trust in the rigor and thoughtfulness of your work.

5.3   Explain

The substance of any well-written Methods section is simply an explanation – a description of *what* you did and *how* you did it. Write logically, organizing the steps of your research in a straightforward way. Keep the style simple: unless a journal's requirements specify otherwise, use first person, favor active verbs, and generally stick to past tense.

Describe your research setting so that readers will recognize how it is similar to or different from their own. Contextual detail is particularly important when describing educational interventions or innovations, organizational initiatives, and quality improvement projects, as readers will need to make judgments about whether or not your findings will transfer to their own settings.

Outline your approach to data collection. Think of the questions readers will have and answer them. How many participants did you recruit? How did you approach recruitment? Was sampling purposive or random? How did you decide when you had sufficient data? Articulate your approach to data analysis. Who was involved and what were their roles? What analytic techniques were used? When the work was collaborative, how were disagreements among team members addressed?

For research involving the use of particular measurement scales or assessment tools, describe these, ideally supported by citations of the literature relating to their development, validation, and use. For exploratory research, give readers some insight into the process. If research involves interviewing participants, give readers a flavor of the kinds of interview prompts that you used. In the following example from an interview study exploring learners' experiences of direct observation during their clinical training, readers are offered critical details about the nature of the interviews that allow them to imagine the process:

> During the interviews, we asked participants to describe the purpose and mechanics of direct observation in their training program, to reflect on their experiences of being observed, and to describe the impact of direct observation on their learning and professional development. Because direct observation takes many forms, we purposefully did not define direct observation for participants, or limit discussion to a particular type of observation. Instead participants were asked to describe the aspects of their work that were typically observed, who observed their work and what form direct observation took (e.g. in-person observation, video, two-way mirror, etc. (LaDonna et al. 2017, p. 500).

Use your explanations strategically to establish yourself as a trustworthy researcher. If you claim to have used theoretical sampling, for example, offer a description of how that actually played out in your study, as opposed to leaving the term dangling. If you decide to make a claim of having "sampled until saturation was reached", tell readers how you defined and operationalized saturation. Sprinkling the *what* and the *how* of explanation with the *why* of justification can be very effective; these two elements should co-exist.

5.4   Educate

Know your audience. Your Methods section needs to make sense for a journal's readership. Consider who comprises that readership and the kind of familiarity – or not – that they have with the work you have done. Jargon can readily infect a Methods section, threatening the accessibility of your work. If your intention is to speak exclusively to an insider audience of researchers who do the same work as you do, then the correct and exacting use of methodological jargon might be critical to establishing your credibility. But much more often, we hope as researchers to reach outside of our own domain, and to encourage uptake of our ideas by those who aren't our insider colleagues. In these cases, we need to interject some education into our explanations.

We frequently conduct constructivist grounded theory research, for example. But we don't assume that the methodology is readily recognized and understood by everyone whom we hope may read our work. Often, then, after identifying our methodology, we'll include a line or two that gently educates. For example:

> Constructivist grounded theory is a rigorous qualitative methodology that is particularly suited to exploring social processes. As constructivists, we hold that knowledge is constructed through interactions between us as researchers, our research participants, and our research setting.

Educating doesn't require that we avoid jargon, but that we attend to defining it for readers so that they can better understand the language we are using. The balance point between illuminating and insulting can be tricky to find when we aim to educate readers, however. Here's where a trusted colleague can help. Find someone who works outside of your research area, but who represents the kind of journal reader you hope to reach, and ask them to read your Methods section and to flag anything they don't understand. You need an individual with the confidence to say "I don't know what this means", so choose your colleague wisely; academics can be surprisingly reluctant to admit when they are baffled, but that's exactly what you need them to do.

5.5   Anticipate

Every methodology has its thorny debates – those issues that reviewers love to seize upon as they critique your work. Savvy methods writing requires you to anticipate those hot button issues and attempt to insulate yourself from the heat they can generate. Anticipating and mitigating controversy may involve carefully choosing your words, or strategically defining a word or phrase to ensure that readers and reviewers don't misinterpret you. Ultimately, your goals are to demonstrate that you are aware of the controversy and to consciously position your work within it. Consider the much-debated issue of "validity" in education research (St. Onge et al. 2017): anticipating this debate, a sophisticated writer will identify where they sit in this methodological conversation, define their approach to validity, and support that approach with credible references.

Exactly where you need to employ an anticipatory strategy can be a moving target. Reviews can be very helpful in revealing evolving rhetorical traps in your field – traps you can avoid next time around. For example, we once received a review of a qualitative Methods section that said "I don't hold with the idea of saturation."

This review planted a red flag around the contested issue of how qualitative researchers decide when they have enough data, and reminded us that the community doesn't always agree on how that process should unfold, how it should be described, or even if it's possible (Varpio et al. 2017). In subsequent papers, we have anticipated this critique, and have handled it in a couple of different ways. Sometimes we have immediately followed our use of the term "saturation" with a sentence or two that shows that we are not naïve to the controversy: e.g., "By 'saturation', we do not mean that further data collection might not have yielded new ideas; rather...". In other cases, we have substituted a different term altogether, such as "sufficiency", which perhaps better reflects the concept of having enough data to craft a coherent analysis, rather than the more implausible notion of having exhausted all possible ideas.

5.6 Reflect

Qualitative researchers are themselves instruments of the research. They shape how data are collected and analyzed, and so they need to engage in reflexivity throughout the research process, considering carefully how their own perspectives, experiences, and identities might influence how they make meaning from their data. And it isn't sufficient for them to keep this process entirely to themselves; a good qualitative Methods section should include more than a passing nod to reflexivity. The researchers should offer some information to readers that helps them to understand the particular perspectives and orientations shaping how the research was conducted.

Reflexivity is no longer the exclusive purview of the qualitative researcher, however. Increasingly, those working in other paradigms are recognizing that reflexivity matters, and are considering how their perspectives shape the questions they ask and the research design choices they make.

An excerpt from a recent paper exploring coaching within medicine and sports offers a nice example of how this reflective process can be represented in a Methods section:

> CW is both an education researcher and an education leader with administrative responsibility for residency training. He identifies as a clinical teacher and as a mentor, but not explicitly as a coach. He has significant musical training. KAL is a scientist with an interest in exploring opportunities to optimize medical training by engaging multiple perspectives – including non-physicians – in teaching and assessment. She identifies as a teacher and as a research supervisor, but not as a mentor or a coach. Both authors are avid sports fans and active participants in recreational sports. Throughout the research process, we reflected on how our interests in, and knowledge about, team and individual sports influenced our analysis. We considered whether our data reinforced or upended our assumptions about coaching and engaged in regular discussions with each other about our evolving perspectives. For example, we were surprised by sports coaches' stronger emphasis on the development of their athletes as people than on their athletic success. Reflecting on how these data challenged our assumptions about sports coaching led us to wonder how such a holistic, learner-centred approach would fit in a patient-centred clinical environment (Watling and LaDonna 2019, p. 470).

This reflection goes beneath the surface of telling the reader who is on the team, and offers insights into how the researchers are oriented to the subject matter they are exploring in both professional and personal terms.

5.7   Conclusion

Advice on writing Methods sections for quantitative researchers tends to remind them that the Methods section is how the validity of their work will be judged. Qualitative researchers may bristle at the notion of "validity" as a measure of the rigor of their work, favoring instead the concept of "trustworthiness." But regardless of the paradigm and its particular language, remember that the Methods section reflects your credibility as a researcher. The Methods section is your chance to say to your reader "Trust me – I know what I'm doing."

And you'd better be convincing.

See One, Do One, Teach One

1. Subject your Methods section to a jargon check. Highlight all the words and phrases that may register as jargon for unfamiliar readers, and ask:

   (a) Do I need to explain this term?
   (b) Am I using the term correctly and consistently?
   (c) Does the term require a citation?

2. Pull out the last set of reviews you received and focus on the reviewers' comments on your Methods section. Can you craft an anticipatory strategy that would pre-empt some of these comments for a similar future study?
3. Draft a reflexivity paragraph for your Methods section. Ask yourself:

   (a) Have I described my background as a researcher/clinician/educator/ person? (as appropriate)
   (b) Have I shared my orientation toward the subject matter?
   (c) Have I described how I enacted these reflections throughout the research process?

References

Kotz, D., & Cals, J. W. L. (2013). Effective writing and publishing scientific papers part IV: Methods. *Journal of Clinical Epidemiology, 66*(8), 817. https://doi.org/10.1016/j.jclinepi.2013. 01.003.

LaDonna, K., Hatala, R., Lingard, L., Voyer, S., & Watling, C. (2017). Staging a performance: Learners' perceptions about direct observation during residency. *Medical Education, 51*(5), 498–510. https://doi.org/10.1111/medu.13232.

St-Onge, C., Young, M., Eva, K. W., & Hodges, B. (2017). Validity: One word with a plurality of meaning. *Advances in Health Science Education, 22*(4), 853–867. https://doi.org/10.1007/s10459-016-9716-3.

Varpio, L., Ajjawi, R., Monrouxe, L. V., O'Brien, B. C., & Rees, C. E. (2017). Shedding the cobra effect: Problematising thematic emergence, triangulation, saturation and member checking. *Medical Education, 51*(1), 40–50. https://doi.org/10.1111/medu.13124.

Watling, C., & LaDonna, K. (2019). Where philosophy meets culture: Exploring how coaches conceptualize their roles. *Medical Education, 53*(5), 467–476. https://doi.org/10.1111/medu.13799.

Chapter 6
Effective Use of Quotes in Qualitative Research

Every qualitative researcher confronts the challenge of selecting the right quotes and integrating them effectively into their manuscripts. As writers we are all guilty of resorting to the default colon as an easy way to tuck quotes into our sentences. And as readers, we have all suffered through papers that read like a laundry list of quotes rather than a story about what the writer learned. This chapter offers suggestions to help you choose the right quotes and integrate them with coherence and style, following the principles of authenticity and argument. To illustrate these suggestions we use a variety of published and created examples; created examples do not have references but include all other conventions of quoted material, including artificial participant numbers (P#).

6.1 Authenticity

At the point of manuscript writing, a qualitative researcher is swimming in sea of data. Innumerable transcript excerpts have been copied and pasted into data analysis software or (for the more tactile among us) onto multi-colored sticky notes. Some of these excerpts we like very much. However, very few of them will make it into the final manuscript, particularly if we are writing for publication in a health research or health professions education journal, with their 3000–4000 word limits.

Selecting the best quotes from among these cherished excerpts is harder than it looks. We should be guided by the principle of authenticity: does the quote offer readers firsthand access to dominant patterns in the data? There are three parts to selecting a good, authentic quote: the quote is illustrative of the point the writer is making about the data, it is reasonably succinct, and it is representative of the patterns in data. Consider this sample quote, introduced with a short phrase to orient the reader:

© The Author(s), under exclusive license to Springer Nature Switzerland AG 2021
L. Lingard, C. Watling, *Story, Not Study: 30 Brief Lessons to Inspire Health Researchers as Writers*, Innovation and Change in Professional Education 19,
https://doi.org/10.1007/978-3-030-71363-8_6

Rather than feeling they were changing identities as they went through their training, medical students described the experience of accumulating and reconciling multiple identities: "the 'life me', who I was when I started this, is still here, but now there's also, like, a 'scientific me' as well as a sort of 'doctor me'. And I'm trying to be all of that. (P15)

This quote is illustrative, providing an explicit example of the point that student identity is multiplying as training unfolds. It is succinct, expressing efficiently what other participants took pages to describe. And it is representative, remaining faithful to the overall sentiments of the many participants reporting this idea.

We have all read – and written! – drafts in which the quoted material does not reflect these characteristics. The remainder of this section addresses these recurring problems.

6.1.1 Is the Quote Illustrative?

A common challenge is the quote that illustrates the writer's point implicitly, but not explicitly. Consider this example:

> Medical students are undergoing a process of identity-negotiation: we're "learning so much all the time, and some of it is the science stuff and some of it is professional or, like, practical ethical things, and we have to figure all that out". (P2)

For this quote to serve as evidence for the point of identity-negotiation, the reader must infer that "figure all that out" is a reference to this process. But readers may read their own meaning into decontextualized transcript extracts. Explicit is better, even if it sacrifices succinctness. In fact, this is the right quote, but we had trimmed away the first three sentences where "figuring out identity" got explicit mention. The quote could be lengthened to include these sentences, or, to preserve succinctness, just that quoted phrase can be inserted into the introduction to the quote:

> Medical students are "figuring out identity", a process of negotiation in which they are "learning so much all the time, and some of it is the science stuff and some of it is professional or, like, practical ethical things, and we have to figure all that out". (P2)

6.1.2 Is the Quote Succinct?

Interview transcripts are characterized by meandering and elliptical or incomplete speech. Therefore, you can search diligently and still come up with a 200-word quote to illustrate your 10-word point. Sometimes the long quote is perfect and you should include it. Often, however, you need to tighten it up. By including succinctness as part of the authenticity principle, my aim is to remind writers to explicitly consider whether their tightening up retains the gist of the quote.

The previous example illustrates one tightening technique: extract key phrases and integrate them into your own, introductory sentence to the quote. Another solution is to use the ellipsis to signal that you have cut part of the quote out:

> Identity formation in the clinical environment is also influenced by materials and tools, "all this stuff you've never used before . . . you don't know where it is or how to use it, and don't even get me started on the computerized record. . . .So many hours and I'm still confused, am I ever going to know where to enter things?" (P7)

The first ellipsis signals that something mid-sentence has been removed. In this case, this missing material was an elaboration of 'all this stuff' that mentioned other details not relevant to the point being made. The second ellipsis follows a period, and therefore signals that at least one sentence has been removed and perhaps more. When using an ellipsis, only remove material that is irrelevant to the meaning of the quote, not material that importantly nuances the meaning of the quote. The goal is not a bricolage that cuts and pastes tiny bits so that participants say what you want them to; it is a succinct-enough representation that remains faithful to the participant's intended meaning.

Changing the wording of a quotation always risks violating the authenticity principle, so writers must do it thoughtfully. Three other situations, however, may call for this approach: to maintain the grammatical integrity of your sentence, to tidy up oral speech, and to translate quoted material into another language. The first is usually not problematic, particularly if you are altering for consistent tense or for agreement of verb and subject or pronoun and antecedent, or replacing a pronoun with its referent. Square brackets signal such changes:

> Interview participants explained that silence was a way of communicating during surgical procedures. Nurses explained that they used silence to "[avoid] direct conflict, like when they ask us for something during the count" (P2) and residents used silence as part of a strategic "wait and see" (P8) approach to avoid "showing that I [don't] know" (P14). (verb tenses changed from past to present)

The second situation can be trickier: when should you tidy up the messiness of conversational discourse? Interview transcripts are replete with what linguists refer to as 'fillers' or 'hesitation markers', sounds and words such as "ah/uh/um/like/you know/right" (Tottie 2016) There is general agreement among qualitative scholars that quotes should be presented verbatim as much as possible, and those engaged in discourse and narrative analysis will necessarily analyze such hesitations as part of the meaning. In other applied social research methodologies, however, writers might do some "light tidying up" both for readability and for ethical reasons, as long as they do not undermine authenticity in doing so (Corden and Sainsbury 2006). Ethical issues include the desire not to do a disservice to participants by representing the um's and ah's of their natural speech, and the concern to protect participant anonymity by removing identifiable linguistic features such as regional or accented speech.

The third situation involves translating data from another language into English. Because most health research is published in English-language journals, this is a pervasive issue; however, it rarely gets explicit attention. In fact, most papers do not acknowledge that data were translated at all. We would argue that, at a minimum, they should do so.

When undertaking translation, researchers need to balance coherence with authenticity. Yes, the quote needs to make sense to readers of English, but the question of what constitutes a valid translation is a matter of some debate. Helmich et al. (2017) explain:

> Researchers within a positivist paradigm may strive for objectivity, trying to reach a 'correct' version of the text, for example by using professional translators and procedures such as forward-backward translation. Scholars adopting a constructivist approach, however, will acknowledge that people who use different languages construct different ways of seeing social life, appreciating that there can be no single correct translation, and that both source and target language always mirror specific cultures and identities. (p. 127)

This is particularly true of metaphors, images, symbols and aphorisms, which interview participants may use liberally in their responses. Conceptual equivalence in such cases is more important than semantic equivalence; in fact, a semantically correct translation is likely to distort the participant's meaning. One way to acknowledge such complexity in translation is to treat translation carefully rather than matter-of-factly, perhaps even presenting both the original text and one or more possible translations to show range of meanings.

Finally, an emerging strategy for succinctness is to put the quotes into a table. Many qualitative researchers resent the constraints of the table format as an incursion from the quantitative realm. However, used thoughtfully, it can offer a means of presenting complex results efficiently. In this example, Goldsmzidt et al. (2012) name, define and illustrate five main types of supervisor interruptions that they observed during their study of case review on internal medicine teaching teams (Fig. 6.1):

Table 1

Types of Supervisors' Interruptions During Patient Case Review Presentations, London Health Sciences Centre, University Hospital, Ontario, Canada, 2010

Type	Description	Example*
Probing for further data	Supervisors ask questions about patient facts, management details, or clarification	Case 17; AM CC-5: Her hemoglobin was 94. A-9: Do we have a previous? CC-5: Yeah, she had one done at the cancer clinic.
Prompting for expected sequence	Supervisors indicate what is expected to come next in the presentation, either proactively or as a correction	Case 10; AM A-3: Cardiovascular exam? IM1-7: Her cardiovascular exam was completely normal.
Teaching around the case	Supervisors teach the team using a variety of teaching styles	Case 2; PM SR-6: So what's the best route to replace potassium? CC-4: Orally. SR-6: Yeah, orally. Do you know why?
Thinking out loud	Supervisors convey their thoughts or provide their interpretation of the case	Case 19; AM A-10: And common things being common, i mean, that probably was the trigger. It'd be highly unlikely that she's got two independent things.
Providing direction	Supervisors give instructions for managing the case	Case 14; AM A-4: He's going to need prolonged IV antibiotics, probably six weeks if he's true osteo and someone's going to need to follow that.

*AM indicates morning case presentation; PM, overnight case presentation; A, attending physician; SR, senior resident; IM1, first-year internal medicine resident; FM1, first-year family medicine resident; and CC, clinical clerk.

Fig. 6.1 Using a tabular format to present quotes

This is a nice example of how "Table 1", conventionally used in quantitative research papers for demographic details of the research sample, can be reconceptualized to feature the key findings from a qualitative analysis. Tables should be supplemented, however, with narrative explanation in which the writer contextualizes and interprets the quoted material. More on this in the section on Argument.

6.1.3   Is the Quote Representative?

We have all been tempted to include the highly provocative quote (that thing we cannot believe someone said on tape), only to realize by the third draft that it misrepresents the data and must be relinquished. Quote selection should reflect strong patterns in the data; while discrepant examples serve an important purpose, their use should be strategic and explicit. Your quote selection should also be distributed across participants, in order that you represent the data set. This may mean using the second- or third-best example rather than continuing to quote the same one or two highly articulate individuals.

As you select quotes to represent main findings, be sure that you retain sufficient context so that readers can accurately infer their meaning. Sometimes this means including the interviewer's question as well as the participant's answer. In focus group research, where the emphasis is on the group discussion, it might be necessary to quote an exchange among participants rather than extracting individual comments. This example illustrates this technique:

Interviewer: And, in your experience, what is it like to participate as a patient storyteller in these orientation sessions for new nurses at the hospital?

P1: Oh, really well, I think it's really important to the nurses, they listen to what we say about our experience and how they can make it better.

Interruption with overlapping talk (both agreement and dissent).

P4: Well, yeah, I agree I usually feel that way. But then there are those days where it's a bit like talking to the wall, like they're waiting for your story to be over with a perma-smile on their faces.

P3: I know what you mean. But I wonder maybe that that's as much about me that day as it is about them. You know, those days when it feels forced, or too raw to be giving up your experience for hospital orientation? (Focus Group 2).

Of course, such a long excerpt threatens the goal of succinctness. Alternatively, you could use multiple quotes from this excerpt in a single sentence of your own:

Some patient storytellers described their role as "really important to the nurses, they listen to what we say about our experience", while others reflected that "there are those days where it's a bit like talking to the wall" or "when it feels forced or too raw". This variability was acknowledged by some to be "as much about me that day as it is about them". (Focus Group 2)

Sometimes a quote is representative but also, therefore, identifiable, jeopardizing confidentiality:

> One participant explained that, "as chair of the competency committee, I prioritize how we spend our time. So that we can pay sufficient attention to this 2nd year resident. She's supposed to be back from maternity leave but she had complications so her rotations need some altering for her to manage." (Clinical Competency Committee 4, P2)

In this (made up) case, the convention of using a legend (Clinical Competency Committee 4, P2) to attribute the quote may be insufficient to protect anonymity. If the study involves few programs and the methods identify them (e.g., Pediatrics and Medicine) and name the institution (e.g., Western University), the speaker may be identifiable to some readers, as may the resident.

6.2   Argument

Even an illustrative, representative quote does not stand on its own: we must incorporate it into our texts, both grammatically and rhetorically. Grammatical incorporation is relatively straightforward, with one main rule to keep in mind: quoted material is subject to the same sentence-level conventions for grammar and punctuation as non-quoted material. Read this example aloud:

> Burnout was experienced by healthcare leaders as well as frontline clinicians, "we all feel at the end of our ropes with the demands of our jobs, to the point where I almost don't care anymore some days". (P7)

Your ear likely hears that this should be two sentences. But quotation marks seem to distract us from this, and we create a run-on sentence by putting a comma between the sentences. An easy correction is to replace the comma with a colon.

> Burnout was experienced by healthcare leaders as well as frontline clinicians: "we all feel at the end of our ropes with the demands of our jobs, to the point where I almost don't care anymore some days". (P7)

Many writers rely on the colon as their default mechanism for integrating quoted material. However, while it is often grammatically accurate, it is not always rhetorically sufficient. That is, the colon doesn't contextualize, it doesn't interpret. Instead, it 'drops' the quote in and leaves the reader to infer how the quoted material illustrates or advances the argument. This is problematic because it does not fulfill the requirement for adequacy of interpretation in presenting qualitative results. As Morrow (2005) argues, "writers should aim for a balance of their interpretations and supporting quotations: an overemphasis on the researcher's interpretations at the cost of participant quotes will leave the reader in doubt as to just where the interpretations came from; an excess of quotes will cause the reader to become lost in the morass of stories" (p. 256).

There are many techniques for achieving this balance between researcher interpretations and supporting quotations. Some techniques retain the default colon but
attend carefully to the material that precedes it. Consider the following examples:

> One clinician said: "Entrustment isn't a decision, it's a relationship". (P21)

> One clinician argued: "Entrustment isn't a decision, it's a relationship". (P21)

> One clinician in the focus group disagreed with the idea that entrustment was about deciding
> trainee progress: "Entrustment isn't a decision, it's a relationship". (P21)

> Focus group participants debated the meaning of entrustment. Many described it matter-of-
> factly as "the process we use to decide whether the trainee should progress", while a few
> argued that "entrustment isn't a decision, it's a relationship". (P21)

These examples offer progressively more contextualization for the quote. The
first example simply drops the quote in following the nondescript verb, "said",
offering no interpretive gloss and therefore exerting minimal rhetorical control
over the reader. The second offers some context via the verb "argued", which
interprets the participant's positioning or tone. The third interprets the meaning of
the quote even more by situating it in the context of a focus group debate. And the
fourth eschews the default colon entirely, integrating two quotes into the narrative
structure the author's sentence to illustrate the dominant and the discrepant positions
on entrustment in this focus group debate.

Integrating quotes into the narrative structure of your sentence, like the last
example, offers two advantages to the writer. First, it interprets the quote for the
reader and therefore exerts strong rhetorical control over the quote's meaning.
Second, it offers variety and style. If your goal is compelling prose, variety and
style should not be underestimated. We have all had the experience of reading
Results sections that proceed robotically: point-colon-quote, point-colon-quote,
point-colon-quote …. If only to make the reader's experience more enjoyable,
your revision process should involve converting some of these to integrated
narration.

Notwithstanding the goal of succinctness, sometimes you will include a longer
quote because it beautifully illustrates the point. However, a long quote may offer
opportunities for readers to focus on images or phrases other than those you
intended, therefore creating incoherence in the argument you are making about
your results. To guard against this, you might try the "quotation sandwich" technique (Graff and Birkenstein 2018) of both an introductory phrase that sets up the
context of the quote and a summary statement following it that emphasizes why you
consider it important and what you are using it to illustrate.

Finally, how many quotes do you need to support your point? More is not
necessarily better. One quote should be sufficient to illustrate your point. Some
points in your argument may not require a quoted excerpt at all. Consider this
example, in which the first sentence presents a finding that is not illustrated with a
quotation:

> Physicians described themselves as being always tired. However, their perceptions of the impact of their fatigue varied, from "not a factor in the care I provide" (P8) to "absolutely killing me…I'm falling asleep at the bedside". (P15)

The finding that physicians are always tired does not require illustration. It is readily understandable and will not surprise anyone; therefore, following it with the quote "I'm tired all the time" (P2) will feel redundant. The second part of the finding, however, benefits from illustration to show the variety of perception regarding impact.

If you do use multiple quotes to illustrate a point in your argument, then you must establish the relations between them for the reader. You can do this between the quoted excerpts or after them, as modelled above with the four examples used to illustrate progressively stronger quote contextualization.

6.3 Conclusion

Quotes can be the life's blood of your qualitative research paper. However, they are the evidence, not the argument. They do not speak for themselves and readers cannot infer what you intend them to illustrate. The authenticity principle can help you select a quote that is illustrative, succinct and representative, while the argument principle can remind you to attend to the grammatical and the rhetorical aspects of integrating the quote into the story you are telling about your research.

See One, Do One, Teach One

1. Check your quotes for Authenticity:

   (a) Does it illustrate explicitly the point you're trying to make?
   (b) Is it as succinct as possible? Can you trim longer quotes? Could you try a table?
   (c) Is it representative? Are there any 'outlier' quotes you should relinquish?

2. Check your quotes for Argument:

   (a) Circle each colon you have used to introduce a quotation from your data. Select some for revision to strengthen the contextualization of the quote. For instance, try to convert some of them to narrative integration rather than setting them off.
   (b) Are any of the quotes unnecessary?
   (c) Where you have used more than one quote to support or develop a point, ensure that you explicitly guide the reader through them with your own text.

References

Corden, A., & Sainsbury, R. (2006). *Using verbatim quotations in reporting qualitative social research: Researchers' views*. York: Social Policy Research Unit.

Goldsmzidt, M., Aziz, N., & Lingard, L. (2012). Taking a detour: Positive and negative impacts of supervisor interruptions during admission case review. *Academic Medicine, 87*(10), 1382–1388. https://doi.org/10.1097/ACM.0b013e3182675b08.

Graff, G., & Birkenstein, C. (2018). *"They say/I say": The moves that matter in academic writing* (4th ed.). New York: W. W. Norton &.

Helmich, E., Cristancho, S., Diachun, L., & Lingard, L. (2017). How would you call this in English?' Being reflective about translations in international, cross-cultural qualitative research. *Perspectives on Medical Education, 6*(2), 127–132. https://doi.org/10.1007/s40037-017-032.

Morrow, S. L. (2005). Quality and trustworthiness in qualitative research in counseling psychology. *Journal of Counselling Psychology, 52*(2), 250–260. https://doi.org/10.1037/0022-0167.52.2.250.

Tottie, G. (2016). Planning what to say: Uh and um among the pragmatic markers. In G. Kaltenbock, E. Keizer, & A. Lohmann (Eds.), *Outside the clause: Form and function of extra-clausal constituents* (pp. 97–122). Amsterdam: John Benjamins Publishing.

Chapter 7
Writing a Discussion
That Realizes Its Potential

A few years ago one of our research teams got a "Major Revision" response from a journal after our manuscript was reviewed. The main critique was that "the Discussion does not realize the potential of the Introduction". That critique sums up beautifully the purpose of a Discussion section: it must bring to fruition the story that the Introduction started. But how can we ensure that our Discussions succeed in this aim?

7.1 Telling the Story

Together, the Introduction and Discussion sections of a manuscript *tell the story*, while the Methods and Results sections *report the study* (Lingard and Watling 2016). For a manuscript to tell a coherent story, its Discussion section ought to provide the '*so what?*', the climax of the work. Often, however, the Discussion falls short in one of two ways. First, we can settle for insipid Discussions that merely summarize results, confess limitations, and suggest future research. This tendency reflects a well-worn 'formula' but it fails to create any narrative arc in the story, leaving much room for improvement and artistry. Or, we can create overly dramatic Discussions, which over-interpret study results with speculation and grand claims (Docherty and Smith 1999). The trick of an effective Discussion is to find the sweet spot between these two poles: a Discussion that tells a story based on the results and places that story into a wider context of knowledge about the problem, but does not overreach.

Resources exist to help writers structure a Discussion section, but they tend towards checklists of items which may not help with the creating of a sense of story in the paper. For instance, the Consort Checklist for randomized trials directs writers to focus their Discussion on three issues: Limitations, Generalizability and Interpretation (CONSORT 2010). Similarly, standards for reporting qualitative health research outline two standards writers should observe for a Discussion section (O'Brien et al. 2014):

> Standard 18: Integration with prior work, implications, transferability, and contribution(s) to the field – Short summary of main findings; explanation of how findings and conclusions connect to, support, elaborate on, or challenge conclusions of earlier scholarship; discussion of scope of application/generalizability; identification of unique contribution(s) to scholarship in a discipline or field.

> Standard 19: Limitations – Trustworthiness and limitations of finding.

Standard 18 in particular offers a helpful list of possible items for inclusion in a Discussion, but writers may still find themselves struggling to move from list to story. This chapter offers two strategies writers can use to make this shift: 1) Think of your ideas as characters in a drama, and carefully consider how to shape their story arcs, and 2) Create a recognizable storyline linking your Introduction and Discussion.

7.2 Who Are Your Main Characters?

A drama metaphor can help you to identify, position and develop the characters in your research story. In suggesting this metaphor, we are not advocating an overly 'dramatic' style of writing. Rather, we are offering a heuristic for clarifying the story you're telling and ensuring that ideas *develop* in the Discussion.

Think of the introduction of your paper as the opening act of a play, and each idea you introduce as a character. How many characters are you bringing on stage? Is the main character clearly indicated? Imagine a manuscript about assessing student professionalism that introduces the following characters in the opening paragraphs: professionalism, ethics, assessment, clerkship, dilemmas, competency, observation, feedback and role modelling. This stage is too full! Pare down the characters, introduce them carefully and ensure that the main character(s) stand out clearly and supporting characters are put in their place. Now, think of the Discussion as Act III, the climax of the story. Which of your supporting characters must return? What will happen to the main character(s) so that they develop? Have you introduced a new main character in the Discussion, or killed off the main character? Both of these are abrupt departures from the conventional storylines in a research manuscript – not impossible, but only to be done purposefully and carefully.

7.3 What's Your Storyline?

As the drama metaphor emphasizes, the Introduction and Discussion are in partnership. You can think of their relationship as a storyline that influences when characters appear and how they develop. In our experience, three storylines recur in health research manuscripts: Coming Full Circle, Deep Exploration and Surprise Insight. Learning to recognize these storylines can help writers to assess the conventions of the journal they're targeting and the affordances of particular storylines for their manuscript.

7.3.1   Coming Full Circle

In a Coming Full Circle storyline, each idea/character presented in the Introduction returns in the Discussion. No new characters are introduced in the Discussion, as all relevant concepts and literatures have been set out in the Introduction and are revisited methodically in the Discussion. This storyline is signaled by few or no new keywords or references in the Discussion section of the paper.

Coming Full Circle is a common structure in quantitative and experimental research manuscripts, where research designs focus on a defined research question. For instance, in a paper describing a randomized controlled trial of two resident duty hours models in critical care, the Introduction presented the main characters/issues of physician fatigue, patient safety, duty hours and care continuity, and the Discussion revisited each of these while interpreting study results in light of the literature (Parshuram et al. 2015). The difference between Coming Full Circle and the tired Discussion 'formula' is the building of this purposeful storyline between the Introduction and Discussion. Rather than just recapping results – reintroducing the main characters from the Intro – they are put in a wider context. The Discussion returns to the characters we met in the Introduction and tells us something more about them as a result of the work.

7.3.2   Deep Exploration

In a Deep Exploration storyline, the Discussion selectively explores a subset of ideas from the Introduction. In this storyline, the main character in the Discussion is not new; it will have been presented in the Introduction. However, new supporting characters may be brought on stage in the Discussion as part of the Deep Exploration of this character's world. This will be signaled by new keywords and references in the Discussion section.

In Deep Exploration storylines, the first paragraph of the Discussion will often provide a brief review of the full company of ideas/characters presented in the Introduction, before diving into one or two in more extensive detail. We expect that many health research and health professional education journals have a (largely tacit) expectation of a Coming Full Circle manuscript structure. Writers can satisfy this expectation by using the first paragraph of the Discussion to review the entire cast before zooming in to focus the Discussion on a few key characters.

Deep Exploration is a common storyline in social sciences research writing generally and health professions education manuscripts specifically. For instance, in a paper describing the development of an observation tool to measure team communication, the Introduction presented the main characters of team communication, communication failure, improvement initiatives, and performance measurement; the Discussion, however, focused mostly on performance measurement, detailing in particular the tradeoffs between reliability and authenticity (Lingard et al. 2006). Deciding that a character deserves a Deep Exploration is a matter of judgment, usually in situations where you *could* come full circle but to do so you would have to confine a character that is straining for more space on stage. Sometimes this becomes clear because you realize, while writing, that readers are going to want more on this character – their curiosity will be piqued, or their assumptions challenged in a way that requires thorough unpacking. You can of course decide to confine that character to the same allotment of spotlight as all the others, and this may be necessary in journals where Coming Full Circle is a strict convention. However, when you can develop one character beyond the others without creating a sense of unexplained imbalance (i.e., without the reader wondering why the other characters are flat), the Deep Exploration storyline is an effective structure to employ.

7.3.3 Surprise Insight

In a Surprise Insight storyline, the Discussion introduces new ideas or main characters that were not presented in the Intro. Sometimes this new idea will be briefly foreshadowed in the Introduction – picture a hooded character who slowly crosses the stage but does not speak – and other times it emerges as entirely new in the Discussion. Surprise Insight storylines include many new references in the Discussion, often from literatures not broached in the Introduction as the writer elaborates the world of this new character.

Surprise Insight storylines are rare in health research, but more likely in qualitative and constructivist research manuscripts, where the research approach invites emergent twists and turns not imagined at the study outset. For example, in a paper from our healthcare teamwork research, the Introduction spotlighted the main characters of inter-professional care, collaboration and leadership. The Discussion summarized the key finding of a double bind for physicians navigating the competing values of leadership and collaboration, and then explicitly introduced a new suite of characters that were necessary to understand this double bind:

> To explore this provocative explanation for our findings, we briefly consider three of the broader systems that support physicians' privileged status: the education system, the health care delivery system, and the medical-legal system. (Lingard et al. 2012, 1765)

The bulk of the Discussion elaborated these new characters. As this example demonstrates, such explicit signposting – "this provocative explanation for our findings" – is critical in a Surprise insight storyline, in order to minimize the chance that the reader may perceive a random detour.

This example illustrates another important point: Surprise Insight is not a reference to new or surprising results. Rather, it is a reference to a new character in the story told about the results. Many studies report new results, but this is not what is meant by a Surprise Insight storyline. Results are study, not story. A Surprise Insight storyline represents a decision to reveal some of the characters in the story in the Discussion rather than putting them all up front in the Intro. That is, because of the results (which may or may not have been surprising themselves), we now have a new way of seeing the problem than the way we set it up in the Introduction. In this case, it is the new way of seeing, the "provocative explanation" of the results in the example above, that is a surprise, not the results themselves. Thus, the Surprise Insight storyline can be particularly effective when the writer wants readers to experience a shift in their perspective, coming to see the problem very differently at the end of the paper than they did at the start.

Writers have some choice of storylines, but their choice must be guided by the conventions of the journal they wish to publish in. Consider questions such as: Will the journal expect symmetry of ideas between Introduction and Discussion? Does the journal allow new references in the Discussion? Will you need to foreshadow an idea in the Introduction or can it appear as new in the Discussion? Read papers in the journal to analyze the relationship between Introductions and Discussions, so that you can learn which storylines are common and discover adaptations of these structures.

7.4 Conclusion

Using the drama metaphor and storyline structure requires writers to shed the notion that the Introduction should represent what was known before the study was launched and the Discussion what is known after it is completed. A good story is rarely chronological, and good academic writers understand that readers do not need to come to understanding in the same stepwise (and sometimes painful!) manner that the researcher did. With this in mind, think about which characters should appear in your Intro/Act I, whether and how they need to reappear in your Discussion/Act III, or which new characters need introduction at this point to strengthen the narrative arc of the story.

Your research study – its methods and results – needs to be reported fully and accurately. Your research story, however, should be told as persuasively as possible. The story you set up in the Introduction needs to develop in the Discussion, based on the results of your work. As a *BMJ* commentary on the subject of effective Discussions put it, "every paper must reach a conclusion that is not contained in its results" (Skelton and Edwards 2000, 1269). The Discussion is the bridge that gets you to that conclusion.

See One, Do One, Teach One

1. Consider your Introduction and Discussion together, and create an inventory of the "characters" (key ideas) in your story. Identify whether each is a main character or a supporting character. Paying particular attention to your supporting characters, consider carefully whether each plays a necessary role. Could any characters be eliminated without losing the plot? Do any supporting characters need to be elevated to main players?

2. Create a 'Storyline' table. In the first column, list all the key ideas (characters) that appear in your introduction. In the next column, put a checkmark if those characters reappear in the Discussion. In the third column, put an asterisk if those characters develop meaningfully when they reappear. Now step back and ask yourself:

   (a) That character that never reappears in the Discussion: does it really need to be in the Intro, or could it be dropped? Does it need to feature in the Discussion?

   (b) That character that appears in the Discussion but NOT in the Intro: How can you prepare the reader for that? Do you intend it to be a surprise, or should it be foreshadowed? Will the surprise work, or might it seem like either a detour or a holding back of key information?

   (c) Those characters that reappear in the Discussion but don't develop: how can you deepen the story to use the results to say something more meaningful about them?

3. Try a Surprise Insight approach to a Discussion section. Ask a friendly reader to tell you if it works. If it doesn't, revise by inserting the relevant characters into the Introduction so that the surprise factor is removed.

References

CONSORT. (2010). *Checklist for reporting randomized trial.* http://www.consort-statement.org/. Accessed 7 Aug 2020.

Docherty, M., & Smith, R. (1999). The case for structuring the discussion of scientific papers. *BMJ, 318,* 1224–1225. https://doi.org/10.1136/bmj.318.7193.1224.

Lingard, L., & Watling, C. (2016). It's a story, not a study: Writing an effective research manuscript. *Academic Medicine, 91*(12), e12. https://doi.org/10.1097/ACM.0000000000001389.

Lingard, L., Regehr, G., Espin, S., & Whyte, S. (2006). A theory-based instrument to evaluate team communication in the operating room: Balancing measurement authenticity and reliability. *BMJ Quality and Safety, 15*(6), 422–426. https://doi.org/10.1136/qshc.2005.015388.

Lingard, L., Vanstone, M., Durrant, M., Fleming, C., Lowe, M., Rashotte, J., et al. (2012). Conflicting messages: Examining the dynamics of leadership on interprofessional teams. *Academic Medicine, 87*(12), 1762–1767. https://doi.org/10.1097/ACM.0b013e318271fc82.

O'Brien, B. C., Harris, I. B., Beckman, T. J., Reed, D. A., & Cook, D. A. (2014). Standards for reporting qualitative research. *Academic Medicine, 89*(9), 1245–1251. https://doi.org/10.1097/ACM.0000000000000388.

Parshuram, C., Friedrich, J., Amaral, A. C., Ferguson, N. D., Baker, G. R., Etchells, E. E., et al. (2015). Patient safety, resident wellbeing and continuity in three resident duty schedules in ICU: A randomized trial. *CMAJ, 187*(5), 321–329. https://doi.org/10.1503/cmaj.140752.

Skelton, J. R., & Edwards, S. J. L. (2000). The function of the discussion section in academic medical writing. *BMJ, 320*, 1269–1270. https://doi.org/10.1136/bmj.320.7244.1269.

Chapter 8
The Art of Limitations

There is no such thing as the perfect research design – at least, not in practice. Research inevitably involves a series of compromises among the principles of rigor, ethics and feasibility. Therefore, a hallmark of a high-quality research manuscript is a section that explicitly attends to how such compromises shape the knowledge the work produces and limit its applicability to the broader domain.

That sounds pretty straightforward, doesn't it? However, many Limitations sections are insufficient, vague, or even misleading. And even though these sections tend to be brief (often treated as afterthoughts in the writing process), they deserve close attention because of their role in the current "medical misinformation mess" (Ioannidis et al. 2017). According to Ioannidis, a preeminent metascience scholar and critic of sloppy science, the mess arises because the reliability of much research evidence is unclear, clinical readers are unable to critically assess its quality or applicability to their context, and, consequently, patients and families lack reliable information to support decision-making. A good Limitations section would help this situation, but many papers are lacking here: Ioannidis' analysis of 400 papers published in leading medical journals found that only 17% used at least one word related to limitations, and none of the 400 papers discussed limitations in the terms of implications for conclusions (Ioannidis 2007). A surprising statistic, to say the least, since a shoddy or nonexistent Limitations section often threatens publication, suggesting as it does that the writer may be naïve about their science.

Even when researchers know intimately the strengths and weaknesses of their own work, they may not fully disclose these in their Limitations sections. Why? Part of the explanation is the rhetorical context of manuscript review: writers perceive a "transparency threshold" (Puhan et al. 2012) beyond which the probability of manuscript acceptance drops sharply. In this chapter, we review three common approaches that health research writers tend to take to the Limitations section. While we acknowledge the rhetorical motivations underpinning each approach, only one of them fulfills the purpose of a Limitations section: to equip readers to judge for themselves the credibility of the results and the applicability of the

L. Lingard, C. Watling, *Story, Not Study: 30 Brief Lessons to Inspire Health Researchers as Writers*, Innovation and Change in Professional Education 19, https://doi.org/10.1007/978-3-030-71363-8_8

conclusions to the reader's context. This chapter ends with a five-step process writers can use to identify, present, and organize their Limitations to successfully achieve this purpose.

8.1   Three Approaches to Limitations

We have identified three common ways that health researchers approach their Limitations sections: The Confession, The Dismissal, or The Reflection. Below we define and illustrate each of these approaches, and consider what motivates them.

8.1.1   The Confession

In The Confession, the writer asks readers to forgive the flaws in study design. Take this example of a common statement, for instance:

> Data collection occurred in a single institutional setting due to limited study resources. Participants who agreed to respond to the survey may represent a biased sample.

The Confession admits the study flaw but does not provide any critical consideration of *why* the design decision was made. "Limited study resources" is an excuse, not a critical consideration, and "may represent a biased sample" is an admission but not a reflection on what this means for the results. The Confession enacts the assumption that the writer will be rewarded for recognizing their study flaws – better to point them out yourself than to have reviewers think you aren't aware of them. But simply stating the compromises made in the study design is insufficient if the Limitations section is going to do its job of indicating how those decisions impact the results and limit the conclusions.

8.1.2   The Dismissal

In The Dismissal, the writer acknowledges concerns only to dismiss their importance. Consider this example of dismissing a well-recognized weakness of observational research:

> Observational research can produce Hawthorne effect, in which participants alter their naturalistic behavior due to the observer's presence. However, we are confident that the practices described in our study represent a robust range of possible strategies that faculty providing clinical feedback to trainees might realistically employ.

Writers taking this approach are recognizable by this admit/dismiss pattern. Yes, the sample size is small, but we are confident it includes the major points of view. Okay, the statistical tests were a fishing expedition, but our p value was significant.

The Dismissal likely arises from the experience that journal reviewers use identified limitations as a basis for rejecting manuscript submissions, so the writer needs to convincingly argue that none of the limitations are fatal.

While you may wish to reassure the reader that the study's strengths provide a counterbalance to a weakness, this is distinct from *dismissing* the weakness. Consider this example from a study of surgical practice variation that asked surgeons to comment on surgical approaches they saw in video clips of trainee performance:

> We acknowledge that asking surgeons to make judgments based on decontextualized clips from procedures within their own specialty may seem to amplify the actual variations in practice. To deal with this potential over-representation, we negotiated closely over which moments of variation should be reported in the data. (Apramian et al. 2018, p. 390)

Or this example which reflects on the predominance of residents in the sample for an interview study about feedback:

> Although we included medical students, residents and practicing doctors in our sample, residents accounted for the majority of our participants, thus providing a particular and perhaps limited perspective. We felt, however, that residents were especially likely to be informative, given that feedback is generally more frequent in training than in practice; we also expected that residents would be closer to their sport or music careers, and thus more readily able to relate and reflect upon specific experiences. (Watling et al. 2014, p. 722)

In both of these cases, the writer does not dismiss the problem they have identified in their design. Rather, they offer some insight into how they responded to that problem. They are not saying, "Just trust me, reader", but offering their response to the problem for the reader's consideration.

As we've said, most design decisions are a compromise among rigor, ethics and feasibility; therefore, they are often double-edged. Describing how a design decision is both a limitation and an asset is also a way of moving beyond Dismissal:

> Although the pre-existing dataset utilised in this study has helped to limit the Hawthorne effect, it also limited the investigators' ability to follow-up with participants to develop a better understanding of their experiences with successful or failed control strategies. . . . (Emmerton-Coughlin et al. 2017, p. 1275)

This writer acknowledges that using a pre-existing set of operating room videos offered both an affordance (lessened Hawthorne effect compared to videos created for research purposes) and a drawback (reduced opportunity to interview the participants in the videos about their experience).

8.1.3 The Reflection

As this last example begins to suggest, the most robust form of Limitations is The Reflection. In this approach, the writer lays out the aspects of the research design that create uncertainty about the knowledge contribution, paying attention to the nature of the uncertainty and its implications (Helmich et al. 2015). This reflective stance applies to design issues ranging from the conceptual to the procedural. The following examples illustrate how writers treat this full range of issues by identifying the design decision, naming the limitation it produces, and reflecting on its implications for the results and their application:

> There are a few aspects of the study that may limit transferability to clinical learning outside of the laboratory. First, the researchers tightly controlled the learning experience and the time on task was artificially [controlled]. In real world use of these strategies, direct instruction would likely take considerably less time. Consequently, the participants in this study may have experienced boredom, which could have confounded post-test performance (Leppink 2017). Second, the authors developed the learning and assessment materials and tested them with a small group of novices and experts solely for use in this experimental setting. Thus, the psychometric properties of the materials generated are not available and they could not be reliably exported into a real word classroom. (Steenhof et al. 2019, p. 747)

In this first example, the limitation is one of methodology: due to the choice of an experimental, laboratory-based design, transferability of results to the clinical learning context is in question. Two design decisions are associated with this challenge: the control of the learning experience and the creation of study materials.

In the next example, procedural and technical limitations related to survey response rates and the scope of the study sample are highlighted. Note the use of complex sentence structure: before the semi-colon, the limitation is identified, while after it the implications are considered, often as an elaboration of the consequences of the design decision.

> Limitations of our study include the low survey response rates at two sites; this affects the validity of our results and threatens our conclusions, especially given potential response bias and hindsight bias. Our results may not be generalisable to other training programmes, non-academic institutions, or to specialty ICUs or ICUs with different case mixes or patient populations. Additionally, we only surveyed internal medicine residents; trainees in other specialties or subspecialties, attending physicians and advanced care practitioners may report different experiences. Finally, there is no evidence for direct causality connecting poor handoffs to adverse events. (Santhosh et al. 2019, p. 633)

Interestingly, the final line reflects on a more macro limitation that those previously detailed. The study is interested in the relationship between ward handoffs and adverse events, but evidence is lacking to support this causal relationship. Ideally, the authors would have gone on to reflect on the implications of this final limitation for their work.

8.2   Drafting and Organizing a Robust Limitations Section

Identifying your study limitations is the first step in writing an effective Limitations section. Limitations derive from research design (what you planned to do), research process (what actually happened), and researcher (how you approached the work). Table 8.1 offers a set of reflective questions to help you critically consider each of these domains and identify the limitations that you should discuss:

Table 8.1 Identifying your limitations

Reflective Question	What were the limitations of my research design?	What were the limitations of my research process?	What were the limitations of my research team?
Elements to consider	Methodology	Recruitment	Stance/orientation
	Theoretical framework	Data quality and completeness	Team membership
	Methods/sample/setting	Delay	Language/culture
Examples	*In a study of care transitions, you interviewed patients about their experiences of hospital discharge but not their caregivers.*	*In a study of care transitions, you intended to interview patient and caregiver dyads, but were unable to recruit caregivers.*	*In a study of care transitions, your research team did not include a patient or caregiver's perspective.*
	In a study of physician fatigue, you shortened an existing, validated survey to improve feasibility.	*In a survey study of physician fatigue, your response rate was low, particularly for female respondents.*	*In a study of physician fatigue, you used a biometric definition of fatigue rather than a sociological one.*

Using this method, you will undoubtedly identify multiple limitations that shape your results and their implications for knowledge. Therefore, you need to think about how to organize them. Ask yourself: How consequential are they for the rigor of the study? Has the study accounted for them in some meaningful way? And to what degree are they double-edged (i.e., a limitation that also offers an affordance)? A robust, reflective Limitations section has an organizational logic that readers can follow; it should not read like a randomly ordered list.

Another decision that writers make regarding the presentation of their limitations is whether to take a problem-based or an appreciative orientation. The previous example illustrates the problem-based orientation which is traditionally found in health services research papers. The problem based orientation to limitations says, "Dear reader, here is what makes this work flawed". Each of the four sentences in the previous example began by declaring a problem: "low survey response rates", "may not be generalizable", "we only surveyed", and "there is no evidence". By contrast, the appreciative orientation says "Dear reader, here is what would make this work better". The following example illustrates this orientation, as the authors acknowledge specific ways in which their design could be strengthened.

> Primary rather than secondary data analysis would strengthen a study of how professionals engage in critically reflective practice and how they learn to do so. Research in other indeterminate contexts could help to refine or challenge the assertions made in this study. Other definitions of critical reflection exist; although we purposefully chose our theoretical basis for this study, we acknowledge that many would consider Mezirow's work on the topic to be foundational. We argue that the strengths of this work in fact lie in the careful selection of our definition and our attention to its philosophical roots. This attention to paradigms allowed for careful and purposeful discussion of practical, pedagogical implications. (Ng et al. 2020, p. 318)

This Limitations section begins with the issue of secondary data analysis. However, rather than presenting this as a problem, it is acknowledged that primary data analysis would strengthen the work. Similarly, the authors reflect that their theoretical choices matter but they do not present those choices as a flaw. They are not apologizing for *not* using Mezirow's foundational definition. Rather, they are acknowledging that a choice had to be made, describing the choice they made and considering implications for their work. When using an appreciative orientation, it is important not to slide into a tone of dismissal: you are not 'spinning' the limitation, but indicating why you made the choices you did and how the work could be strengthened. Also, writers must recognize that reviewers may respond to the appreciative approach by wondering, "Yes that would strengthen this work, so why didn't you do it that way in the first place?" Therefore, the best strategy may be to consider which of your identified limitations would be best presented using a problem-based or appreciative orientation, and vary your stance accordingly.

One study cannot do or be everything, so your goal should not be to apologize for everything your study *isn't*. Be explicit about choices, present the thinking behind those choices, and acknowledge their influence on study results and conclusions. Finally, your Limitations should be congruent with your research paradigm. A phenomenological study of first episode schizophrenia experiences in adolescents should not list as a limitation a lack of generalizability, no more than an experimental study of pattern recognition in expert diagnosticians should list as a limitation a failure to iteratively refine the protocol as participants were added to the sample. Keep in mind the principles of rigor relevant to your research paradigm as you think about which of your design decisions constrain the comprehensiveness or quality of your results and, therefore, the implications of your conclusions.

8.3   Conclusion

Of the three approaches we've described, only The Reflection gets to the heart of what a limitations section ought to accomplish: a considered argument about design compromises, the sources of uncertainty they produce in the research, and what these uncertainties mean for how a particular knowledge contribution should be taken up by others. This kind of Limitations section takes more space, but it tends to convey a researcher who is in command of their methodology, recognizes the compromises they have made, and can offer trustworthy guidance to readers on interpreting findings. In short, it should increase your credibility with reviewers and readers, not threaten it.

See One, Do One, Teach One
5 Steps for Drafting a Robust Limitations Section

1. **Identify**: Use Table 1 to create a catalogue of issues that should be discussed in your Limitations section.
2. **Describe**: Present each limitation in detailed but concise terms, including an explanation of why it exists.
3. **Discuss**: Explain what you did to address the limitation or the reasons why the limitation could not be addressed. When possible, cite other studies that confronted similar limitations and compare your response to theirs.
4. **Assess**: Reflect on how each limitation impacts the findings *and* conclusions of your study. Consider how it could point to the need for further research.
5. **Organize**: Decide how you will organize this material, and whether/when you will take a problem-based or an appreciative orientation.

References

Apramian, T., Cristancho, S., Sener, A., & Lingard, L. (2018). How do thresholds of principle and preference influence surgeon assessments of learner performance? *Annals of Surgery, 268*(2), 385–390. https://doi.org/10.1097/SLA.0000000000002284.

Emmerton-Coughlin, H., Schlachta, C., & Lingard, L. (2017). 'The other right': Control strategies and the role of language use in laparoscopic training. *Medical Education, 51*(12), 1269–1276. https://doi.org/10.1111/medu.13420.

Helmich, E., Boerebach, B., Arah, O., & Lingard, L. (2015). Beyond limitations: Improving how we handle uncertainty in health professions education research. *Medical Teacher, 37*(11), 1043–1050. https://doi.org/10.3109/0142159X.2015.1073239.

Ioannidis, J. P. (2007). Limitations are not properly acknowledged in the scientific literature. *Journal of Clinical Epidemiology, 60*(4), 324–329. https://doi.org/10.1016/j.jclinepi.2006.09.011.

Ioannidis, J. P. A., Stuart, M. E., Brownlee, S., & Strite, S. A. (2017). How to survive the medical misinformation mess. *European Journal of Clinical Investigation, 47*(11), 795–802. https://doi.org/10.1111/eci.12834.

Ng, S. L., Mylopoulos, M., Kangasjarvi, E., Boyd, V. A., Teles, S., Orsino, A., et al. (2020). Critically reflective practice and its sources: A qualitative exploration. *Medical Education, 54*(4), 312–319. https://doi.org/10.1111/medu.14032.

Puhan, M. A., Aakl, E. A., Bryant, D., Xie, F., Apolone, G., & ter Riet, G. (2012). Discussing study limitations in reports of biomedical studies: The need for more transparency. *Health and Quality of Life Outcomes, 10*(23). https://doi.org/10.1186/1477-7525-10-23.

Santhosh, L., Lyons, P. G., Rojas, J. C., Ciesielski, T. M., Beach, S., Farnan, J. M., et al. (2019). Characterising ICU-ward handoffs at three academic medical centres: Process and perceptions. *BMJ Quality & Safety, 28*, 627–634. https://doi.org/10.1136/bmjqs-2018-008328.

Steenhof, N., Woods, N. N., Van Gerven, P. W. M., & Mylopoulos, M. (2019). Productive failure as an instructional approach to promote future learning. *Advances in Health Science Education, 24*, 739–749. https://doi.org/10.1007/s10459-019-09895-4.

Watling, C., Driessen, E., van der Vleuten, C. P., & Lingard, L. (2014). Learning culture and feedback: An international study of medical athletes and musicians. *Medical Education, 48*(7), 713–723. https://doi.org/10.1111/medu.12407.

Chapter 9
Bonfire Red Titles

Some time ago Lorelei painted her front door red. The rest of the house was conservative: beige wood siding and white trim on a classic, two-story design. To the neighborhood, it said, 'We are like you; we belong here'. Of course, it also said, 'Nothing particularly exciting is going on behind these walls.' So one morning Lorelei biked to the hardware store, returned with a can of "Bonfire Red" paint and fixed that little bit of false advertising.

A title is like a front door: it serves as advertising for what's inside your research paper. Have a look at the last title you wrote for an academic manuscript. Is it a red door or a white one? Does it draw readers into your work or encourage them to walk by? Academic journals (and edited books, and conference programs) are full of titles that make us want to keep walking. Some are boring, some are obscure, some are cutesy. So many ways to go wrong and the implications are grave. Most of us find the works we read by searching online databases like Google Scholar, so the title is the first thing your prospective readers will see. To ensure it isn't the *last* thing they see, your title needs to be more than an afterthought. This chapter offers strategies to ensure that your title is engaging and informative, memorable and retrievable.

9.1   The Title's Content

The content of your title needs to both attract and inform. First, as journalists say, 'don't bury the lede': the most important idea should be up front, explicit, and memorable. Consider this example:

> The Rising Challenge of Training Physician-Scientists: Recommendations from a Canadian National Consensus Conference. (Strong et al. 2018)

Here, the lede contains important keywords: "training" and "physician-scientists". These keywords ensure that others interested in physician-scientist training

L. Lingard, C. Watling, *Story, Not Study: 30 Brief Lessons to Inspire Health Researchers as Writers*, Innovation and Change in Professional Education 19, https://doi.org/10.1007/978-3-030-71363-8_9

will retrieve your work via online search engines. As this example also shows, however, a good lede has more than keywords; it also signals the 'so what' of the work, in this case "the rising challenge'. Let's look at another example:

> The Myth of Ivory Tower versus Practice-oriented Research: A Systematic Review of Randomized Studies in Medical Education. (Tolsgaard et al. 2020)

Here, keywords such as "medical education" and "research" position this work within a particular conversation. The word "myth" is not a keyword but it signals the purpose and main finding of this work: a challenge to the longstanding assumption that medical education research is polarized between theoretical and applied work.

You may find that there are many keywords of relevance to your work. Choose carefully and help the reader see the relationships among them. This title is packed full of keywords:

> Association Between Physician Burnout and Patient Safety, Professionalism, and Patient Satisfaction: A Systematic Review and Meta-analysis. (Panagioti et al. 2018)

These keywords may all be relevant to the paper, but each references a vast and distinct body of literature. Which is most important? How do they relate to one another? Which conversation is this paper joining? The revision below shifts from the descriptive format of the original to an interrogative format:

> Does Physician Burnout Threaten Patient Safety, Professionalism, and Patient Satisfaction? A Systematic Review and Meta-analysis.

This shift clearly positions physician burnout as the central issue and creates space for a new verb, "threaten". This verb implies the purpose of the work and suggests the relationship between the main keyword and the other three. Admittedly, this version is less 'neutral' than the original, and that neutrality might be important to the authors. Here's a different version:

> Does Physician Burnout Impact Patient Safety, Professionalism, and Patient Satisfaction? A Systematic Review and Meta-analysis.

Toning the verb down from "threaten" to "impact" increases neutrality while still giving a stronger sense of purpose than the original construction.

In addition to the right keywords and a sense of purpose, an effective title has some flair and evokes the tone of the article. Words like "myth" and "threaten" tell us what kind of story the authors will tell in the story. While some health research journals prefer a neutral tone that minimizes authorial voice, neutral shouldn't necessarily be your goal. Play around a bit and see if you can find a tone that is measured but notable. In qualitative papers, an iconic quote can provide flair:

> 'If you can't make it, you're not tough enough to do medicine': A Qualitative Study of Sydney-based Medical Students' Experiences of Bullying and Harassment in Clinical Settings. (Colenbrander et al. 2020)

Opening with the voice of a study participant, this title pulls readers immediately into the context of the work. Writers can also infuse their titles with flair by drawing on metaphor, wordplay or allusion:

A Tea-Steeping or i-Doc Model for Medical Education? (Hodges 2010)

This example uses two metaphors – "tea-steeping" and "i-Doc" – to capture a debate among educators about how training should be organized. The first, "tea-steeping", is now used as short-hand for medical education's traditional assumption that competence arises from learners spending sufficient time in training settings. That's the sign of a successful bit of wordplay: it makes its way into the shared lexicon of the scholarly field. The second metaphor, however, has not had the same uptake, a reminder of the unpredictability of metaphor. Sometimes it sticks, sometimes it doesn't.

To try this yourself, take the central ideas in the conversation you're trying to join and play with them. Are there metaphors that would express an idea evocatively? Can you coin a new phrase that will express an idea in a novel way and be taken up by others? Vet your possibilities carefully with readers to make sure the metaphor, allusion or wordplay resonates in the way you intend. Put it into an online search engine and see what comes up: you don't want to attach your article to the wrong conversation.

While you shouldn't overlook flair, you also shouldn't overdo it. You want your title to advertise your work as exciting *and* credible. The colon title can help balance style and science (Sword 2012), by piquing interest before the colon and establishing credibility after it. Consider this title:

#MeToo in EM: A Multicenter Survey of Academic Emergency Medicine Faculty on their Experiences with Gender Discrimination and Sexual Harassment. (Lu et al. 2020)

With a Twitter hashtag before the colon, this title is catchy and current. What follows the colon, however, emphasizes the science with a description of the methodology and the keywords "gender discrimination" and "sexual harassment". Take care when using popular culture references in titles: popular culture is context-specific and, therefore, potentially meaningless beyond its point of origin. Furthermore, a few years hence, popular culture references can sound passé rather than au courant. A title Lorelei wrote many years ago now makes her wince: "Look Who's Talking: Teaching and Learning Using the Genre of Medical Case Presentations" (Spafford et al. 2006). Why? Because it squanders the lede on a (bad) movie reference that would be obscure to most readers today. It is some comfort to know we're not alone in such faux pas: a study of the use of Bob Dylan references in scientific titles found 135 uses of the phrase, "The times they are a-changin'" (Gornitzki et al. 2015). Assuming that these authors are not aiming to join a scholarly conversation about Dylan, this title phrase is not helping those articles jump to the top of anyone's search results.

It's a small step from catchy to clichéd. During copyediting, a journal once asked us to change a title we thought was quite catchy: "First Do No Harm: An Exploration of Faculty Perspectives on the In-Service Training Evaluation of Residents". The copy editor flagged two problems with the phrase "First do no harm": it unduly emphasized one of multiple findings in the study and it was popular to the point of clichéd. Sure enough: it yields over 300,000 disparate results when typed into the

SpringerLink search engine, and more than 2 million when typed into Google Scholar! We took the advice and dropped the colon structure altogether in the published title: "An exploration of faculty perspectives on the in-training evaluation of residents" (Watling et al. 2010). More pedestrian than the first version, but also more focused and discoverable.

9.2   The Title's Form

Being strategic about your title is easier when you have a variety of models to play with. Structurally and linguistically, scientific titles can be divided multiple ways. At a very basic level, we can distinguish titles that are declarative, descriptive and interrogative (Brabazon 2020). Declarative titles reveal the main finding:

> Later Emergency Provider Shift Hour is Associated with Increased Risk of Admission: A Retrospective Cohort Study. (Tyler et al. 2020)

Descriptive titles identify the central issue and approach:

> A Mixed Methods Study Examining Teamwork Shared Mental Models of Interprofessional Teams during Hospital Discharge. (Manges et al. 2020)

Interrogative titles present the central issue in the form of a question:

> Do In-training Evaluation Reports Deserve their Bad Reputation? A Study of the Reliability and Predictive Ability of ITER Scores and Narrative Comments. (Ginsburg et al. 2013)

More elaborate title taxonomies based on corpus analysis also exist. For instance, Table 9.1 adapts Hartley's 2007 taxonomy of twelve title types using the example of a study of caregiver fatigue. Such taxonomies offer a useful heuristic for encouraging creativity and exploring how your title might accomplish a range of goals.

Another structural distinction is whether you use a colon in your title or not. Colon titles are popular because their structure is tailor-made for the dual 'attract-and-inform' purpose. Before the colon you grab the reader's attention; after it you supply details about geography, temporality, or methodology. Keep in mind, though, that the colon structure invariably tempts you towards longer titles. If your draft title has a colon, try to write it without. Is anything lost? A title without a colon can be powerful; we find when we look back over our publications that they are some of our favorites:

> Stories Doctors Tell. (Moniz et al. 2017)

> Time as a Catalyst for Tension in Nurse-Surgeon Communication. (Espin and Lingard 2001)

> Assessment, Feedback and the Alchemy of Learning. (Watling and Ginsburg 2019)

Table 9.1   12 Title types

Type	Example
Titles that announce a general subject	Caregiver fatigue
Titles that particularize a theme	Caregiver fatigue: a crisis in geriatric mental health
Titles that ask a question	What do caregivers of Alzheimer's patients need to keep going?
Titles that provide an answer	Caregivers need community and respite
Titles that present the author's position	Caregivers: a taken-for-granted resource holding up healthcare
Titles that highlight a research method	Caregiving: a phenomenological exploration
Titles that suggest guidelines or comparisons	The do's, do nots and don't knows of caregiver support
Titles that startle or surprise	Praying for death: Caregiving, vulnerability and complexity at the end of life
Titles that use alliteration	When caregivers can't care: A scoping review of the impacts of caregiver fatigue
Titles that use allusion	Honor thy father and thy mother: Children caregivers
Titles that use puns	Caregiver fatigue and patient safety: A wake up call
Titles that completely mystify	When the lights go out

Adapted from Hartley (2007)

9.3   The Title's Context

Whether titles will work or not has to do with more than just the words you use. Sword (2012) advises to attend not only to the title's text (what is said), but also to its paratext and subtext (what is implied). All three contribute to its impact and effectiveness in a given context. Understanding how they work together may help you to write shorter, punchier titles.

Paratext is any extra-textual matter that accompanies and influences the meaning of a title. In a journal, this includes author names and affiliations, journal name, perhaps the topic of a special issue. Consider this example:

> RCT = Results Confounded and Trivial: The Perils of Grand Educational Experiments. (Norman 2003)

The author of this article is a leading researcher in the medical education field, which adds paratextual meaning to this title. It says, "this title's stance may be playful but the paper is written by a respected researcher and therefore should not be taken lightly". This paratextual dimension may explain why some researchers are reluctant to craft more daring titles; if they do not feel confident in their established ethos in the field, they may feel that work titled playfully could be dismissed as frivolous. Ask a trusted reader to tell you whether a daring title lacks the paratext of credibility: you may need to wait to use it until you are better established in the scholarly conversation.

Subtext is any message in the title that is not stated explicitly in words but can be inferred. The deliciously sacrilegious translation of RCT as "results confounded and trivial" rather than "randomized controlled trial" implies the subtext, "I am sufficiently confident to oppose a dominant scientific assumption". Whether the paper will bear out this subtextual message is another matter, but it is part of what the title advertises to the reader.

Attention to paratext and subtext can help writers be more strategic in the titles they create. Ask yourself, what does the journal context imply? For instance, if you're publishing in *Qualitative Health Research*, then using the phrase "qualitative research study" in your title is likely redundant. Similarly, a colon title that is provocative on one side and conventional on the other can subtextually imply that the work is balanced – both catchy and solid.

9.4 Title Traps to Avoid

Don't write the title quickly, just before submission. Keep a running draft of possibilities and revise them as the work matures, honing until you have the perfect fit. Early titles will likely be 'kitchen sink' versions that include every relevant keyword and methodological marker. As you revise, prune and select what matters most. Think about how subtext and paratext can supply some of what you leave out. Pare away adjectives. Focus on nouns and verbs. Make every word work hard.

Use irony, puns and humor sparingly. Many of us are aiming for an international audience, and these features often don't translate well across cultures. Furthermore, amusing titles may attract less citation than more serious titles (Sagi and Yechiam 2008), suggesting that they may be perceived as less credible. While you want your title to stand out, there is a fine line between flair and frivolity.

Minimize jargon and abstractions. Specialized jargon abounds in academic titles, and while this might serve to signal membership in a scholarly community, it is not always necessary and risks narrowing the readership for your work. Simple and accessible may be better, as the title of this highly cited paper illustrates: "What Every Teacher Needs to Know About Clinical Reasoning" (Eva 2005). There is no jargon in this title. Its claim that the paper includes a message about 'what every teacher needs to know' is reflected in candid and accessible language.

Don't set up expectations the paper can't fulfill. We have had editors tell us that "Your title does not closely enough reflect the work described: please revise to more accurately depict the study's method and results". Such requests are a reminder that 'catchy' and 'nuanced' are difficult to achieve simultaneously, and the writer must balance them artfully.

Don't flout the journal's requirements. When journals offer specific guidelines for titles, writers should try to abide by them. Of course, journals can offer rather contradictory suggestions: they'd like the title to include "all information … that will make electronic retrieval of the article both sensitive and specific", but they also advise that "concise titles are easier to read than long, convoluted ones" (Instructions for Authors 2016). The best way to know if you're balancing the dimensions of a good title is to make a short list of titles and ask readers for feedback: Does the title grab them? Does the paper follow through?

9.5   Conclusion

Your title needs to do three things well: grab the reader's attention, represent the work faithfully, and maximize the work's digital visibility. And, as a general rule, if you can have a bonfire red door rather than a white one, go for it!

> **See One, Do One, Teach One**
> 1. Look through your CV and analyze your titles. Do you have a habitual approach? Is it declarative, descriptive, or interrogative?
> 2. Find the title you like least in your CV. Identify its weaknesses and rewrite it using this chapter's lessons on content and form.
> 3. Put the keywords for your current manuscript draft into Google Scholar or SpringerLink. What titles appear? Will these keywords affiliate you with the right scholarly conversation? If any produce irrelevant hits, reconsider whether they should be featured in your title.
> 4. Keep a draft of possible titles as you work on a research project. Use the taxonomy in Table 1 to stretch your repertoire and refine them as the work matures. Over the life of the project, you may need more than one. Some may be better for conference abstracts than original research papers, but central keywords or coined terms should remain consistent.

References

Brabazon, T. (2020, September 11). *Vlog 234: Titles* [Video]. Youtube. https://www.youtube.com/watch?v=1aw8GkKCbpU&t=

Colenbrander, L., Causer, L., & Haire, B. (2020). 'If you can't make it, you're not tough enough to do medicine': A qualitative study of Sydney-based medical students' experiences of bullying and harassment in clinical settings. *BMC Medical Education, 20*. https://doi.org/10.1186/s12909-020-02001-y.

Editorial Board. Instructions for authors. *Perspectives on Medical Education*. http://www.springer.com/education+%26+language/journal/40037. Accessed 9 Mar 2016.

Espin, S., & Lingard, L. (2001). Time as a catalyst for tension in nurse-surgeon communication. *AORN Journal, 74*(5), 672–682. https://doi.org/10.1016/S0001-2092(06)61766-3.

Eva, K. (2005). What every teacher needs to know about clinical reasoning. *Medical Education, 39*(1), 98–106. https://doi.org/10.1111/j.1365-2929.2004.01972.x.

Ginsburg, S., Eva, K., & Regehr, G. (2013). Do in-training evaluation reports deserve their bad reputations? A study of the reliability and predictive ability of ITER scores and narrative comments. *Academic Medicine, 88*(10), 1539–1544. https://doi.org/10.1097/ACM.0b013e3182a36c3d.

Gornitzki, C., Larsson, A., & Fadeel, B. (2015). Freewheelin' scientists: Citing Bob Dylan in the biomedical literature. *BMJ, 351.* https://doi.org/10.1136/bmj.h6505.

Hartley, J. (2007). There's more to the title than meets the eye: Exploring the possibilities. *Journal of Technical Writing and Communication, 37*(1), 95–101.

Hodges, B. D. (2010). A *tea-steeping* or i-Doc model for medical education? *Academic Medicine, 85*(9), S34–S44. https://doi.org/10.1097/ACM.0b013e3181f12f32.

Lu, D. W., Lall, M. D., Mitzman, J., Heron, S., Pierce, A., Hartman, N. D., et al. (2020). #MeToo in EM: A multicenter survey of academic emergency medicine faculty on their experiences with gender discrimination and sexual harassment. *The Western Journal of Emergency Medicine, 21* (2), 252–260. https://doi.org/10.5811/westjem.2019.11.44592.

Manges, K., Groves, P. S., Farag, A., Peterson, R., Harton, J., & Greysen, S. R. (2020). A mixed methods study examining teamwork shared mental models of interprofessional teams during hospital discharge. *BMJ Quality & Safety, 29*, 499–508. https://doi.org/10.1136/bmjqs-2019-009716.

Moniz, T., Lingard, L., & Watling, C. (2017). Stories doctors tell. *JAMA, 318*(2), 124–125. https://doi.org/10.1001/jama.2017.5518.

Norman, G. (2003). RCT = results confounded and trivial: The perils of grand educational experiments. *Medical Education, 37*(7), 582–584. https://doi.org/10.1046/j.1365-2923.2003.01586.x.

Panagioti, M., Geraghty, K., Johnson, J., Zhou, A., Panagopoulou, E., Chew-Graham, C., et al. (2018). Association between physician burnout and patient safety, professionalism, and patient satisfaction: A systematic review and meta-analysis. *JAMA Internal Medicine, 178*(10), 1317–1331. https://doi.org/10.1001/jamainternmed.2018.3713.

Sagi, I., & Yechiam, E. (2008). Amusing titles in scientific journals and article citation. *Journal of Information Science, 34*(5), 680–687. https://doi.org/10.1177/0165551507086261.

Spafford, M. M., Schryer, C. F., Mian, M., & Lingard, L. (2006). Look who's talking: Teaching and learning using the genre of medical case presentations. *Journal of Business and Technical Communication, 20*(2), 121–158. https://doi.org/10.1177/1050651905284396.

Strong, M. J., Busing, N., Goosney, D., Harris, K., Horsley, T., Kuzyk, A., et al. (2018). The rising challenge of training physician–scientists: Recommendations from a Canadian national consensus conference. *Academic Medicine, 93*(2), 172–178. https://doi.org/10.1097/ACM.0000000000001857.

Sword, H. (2012). *Stylish academic writing.* Cambridge, MA: Harvard University Press.

Tolsgaard, M. G., Kulasegaram, K. M., Woods, N., Brydges, R., Ringsted, C., & Dyre, L. (2020). The myth of ivory tower versus practice-oriented research: A systematic review of randomised studies in medical education. *Medical Education.* https://doi.org/10.1111/medu.14373.

Tyler, P. D., Fossa, A., Joseph, J. W., et al. (2020). Later emergency provider shift hour is associated with increased risk of admission: A retrospective cohort study. *BMJ Quality & Safety, 29*, 465–471. https://doi.org/10.1136/bmjqs-2019-009546.

Watling, C. J., & Ginsburg, S. (2019). Assessment, feedback and the alchemy of learning. *Medical Education, 53*(1), 76–85. https://doi.org/10.1111/medu.13645.

Watling, C. J., Kenyon, C. F., Schulz, V., Goldszmidt, M. A., Zibrowski, E., & Lingard, L. (2010). An exploration of faculty perspectives on the in-training evaluation of residents. *Academic Medicine, 85*(7), 1157–1162. https://doi.org/10.1097/ACM.0b013e3181e19722.

Chapter 10
Making Every Word Count:
Keys to a Strong Research Abstract

'Abstract' is one of those curious English words – like 'sanction' or 'cleave' – that can represent near-opposite ideas, depending on context. When we think of abstract art, for example, we don't typically imagine a clear and precise representation of an identifiable subject; in fact, we often wonder if we have interpreted the meaning of the piece as the artist had intended. But a research abstract must represent our work clearly and precisely. We can't afford to leave readers with a range of possible interpretations. In this chapter, we consider the purpose of a research abstract and the methods we might use to craft a strong one.

10.1   Purpose and Audience

Abstracts function within two main contexts: paper abstracts, which accompany full manuscripts, and conference abstracts, which typically stand alone. Regardless of context, abstracts serve a dual purpose. First, they accurately summarize the work, so readers know what it is about. Second, they act as what Varpio et al. (2016) call "promotional documents", aiming to persuade the reader that the work is worthy of their attention.

A high-quality abstract not only describes the work in a straightforward and informative manner, but also includes the keywords that will draw the attention of those working in the same and related fields. Think about your intended audience, and about the words they will enter into a search engine to find papers germane to their work. Consider including keywords that your title couldn't accommodate, to strengthen linkages with relevant domains. The abstract offers a golden opportunity to put your work on the right maps. Make the most of it.

The reach and impact of your work hinges not only on the clarity and the accessibility of the abstract, but also on its persuasiveness. Journal editors may use the abstract to filter submitted manuscripts, sometimes making the decision to reject

L. Lingard, C. Watling, *Story, Not Study: 30 Brief Lessons to Inspire Health Researchers as Writers*, Innovation and Change in Professional Education 19, https://doi.org/10.1007/978-3-030-71363-8_10

the paper based on the abstract alone (Groves and Abbasi 2004). Once the paper is published, the abstract's screening function continues. Readers typically start with the abstract, using it to determine whether a paper is relevant to their goals. Researchers decide, based on the abstract, if the paper belongs in their literature search, and ultimately if the work will be cited. For conference abstracts, the stakes are similarly high: access to the speaker's podium depends on the abstract alone and its ability to convince reviewers that the work deserves exposure. And even after the abstract is accepted for presentation at the conference, its work isn't done. Conference participants will vote with their feet, using abstracts to help them decide which presentations to attend.

Good abstracts are invitations: they invite readers to engage with your paper, and conference goers to engage with your presentation. Like invitations, they should create a sense of anticipation, while ensuring that their promises are accurate and trustworthy.

10.2   Getting Started

Many of us labor over the manuscript, subjecting it to multiple rounds of painful revisions before finally feeling like the paper is ready to send to a journal. And then just as we are poised to hit "submit", we remember that the paper still needs an abstract. Deflated, we try to throw something acceptable together so we can get the paper off our desk. Sound familiar?

There's nothing inherently wrong with leaving the abstract until late in the writing process. Cook and Bordage (2016) recommend, in fact, that the abstract be written last, only after the paper is already complete. Their sound rationale is that this approach ensures that the abstract matches the paper – that you summarize what you actually said, rather than what you thought you might say. Writing the abstract last, though, shouldn't mean that the abstract is an afterthought. Crafting something that is at once brief, comprehensive, and convincing is no easy task. Budget time for it, and don't underestimate the effort that will be required to get the abstract just right.

For conference abstracts, we often don't have the luxury of having a complete paper already written that we can draw from. Challenging as it may be to write an accurate summary of work that doesn't yet exist in manuscript form, the exercise can be a useful one. Writing an abstract often brings focus and precision to a developing research story; it may even make the subsequent manuscript writing easier. Just be sure, in those situations where a conference presentation becomes a paper, that you don't simply reuse the conference abstract. Modify and refine the early abstract so that it accurately represents the final manuscript.

In approaching abstract writing, start by consulting the "Instructions for Authors" section of the website of your target journal, or the conference abstract guidelines, looking specifically for their required abstract style. Few other parts of your submission will be as tightly controlled; you are likely to have a word count maximum that you should view as firm, and a required template. That template may be structured, with required subheadings like Purpose/Background, Methods, Results, and Conclusions, or may be unstructured, requiring a single paragraph describing the study. Even for unstructured abstracts, the writing should be logical and organized, ticking essentially the same boxes as a structured abstract.

10.3 Telling a Convincing Story

The Problem/Gap/Hook heuristic is particularly useful for abstracts, given their compressed nature. The advantage of this heuristic is that it helps to ensure that everything you put in the abstract forms a purposeful part of a scientific story. Unlike the main text of the paper, where persuasive arguments can be developed over several paragraphs, the abstract requires you to get right to the heart of things. Aim for a strong opening sentence that wastes little time on platitudes like "Medicine is a calling to care" or "Assessments shape learning". What you want to open with is a problem to which readers will immediately relate. Consider the opening sentence of this abstract, from a seminal paper on the treatment of malignant brain tumours:

> Glioblastoma, the most common primary brain tumor in adults, is usually rapidly fatal (Stupp et al. 2005).

As a reader, one can't help but snap to attention with an opening salvo like this one. The problem is unambiguous, the disruption immediate.

One can be effective without being quite so blunt, especially if the journal is a bit more generous with its word count. But readers shouldn't have to work to figure out what problem motivated the study. In the following example, there's a brief "topic" sentence before the problem is revealed:

> Feedback conversations play a central role in health professions workplace learning. However, learners face a dilemma: if they engage in productive learning behaviours (such as asking questions, raising difficulties, offering opinions or contesting ideas), they risk exposing their limitations or offending the educator (Johnson et al. 2020).

Notice, though, that the topic sentence is not mere filler. Instead of settling for a mundane opener like "Feedback is of critical importance in health professions education", the authors use this sentence to state their orientation toward feedback (feedback as conversation) and to identify their specific setting (workplace learning). And then they immediately zero in on a problem, using the word "dilemma" as a helpful signpost, just in case a reader was inclined to miss it.

Once the problem is pinpointed, use the remaining one or two sentences of the opening section of the abstract – the "Purpose" or "Background" section – to call out the gap in the current understanding of that problem that your study will fill. Cut to the chase; the abstract is not the place to spend 3–4 sentences demonstrating that you have read the literature. A single, complex sentence can sometimes facilitate the concise articulation of a gap, as in this sentence from the abstract of a paper exploring faculty perspectives on curriculum change:

> Although there is substantial literature on the critical role of leadership in successful curricular change, the voices of frontline faculty teachers implementing such change have not been explored (Venance et al. 2014).

Using a hook in your abstract advances its promotional function. In a full paper, the hook might appear in two places: as a promise in the introduction (i.e. "If we better understand x, then we can be more effective at y. . ."), and as an implication in the Discussion ("Our work has a number of implications for the field. . ."). Abstracts rarely afford the luxury of reinforcing the hook in this way, and so the best strategy is often to highlight the hook in the Conclusions section, which will leave the reader with the strongest impression. Be clear and unambiguous, rather than making readers guess what your work means (Cook and Bordage 2016). As Schimel (2012) cautioned, "Don't blow the punchline." Consider this concluding piece of an abstract from a study exploring how medical students conceptualize fatigue:

> Despite empirical evidence to the contrary, the prevailing assumption amongst our participants is that an ability to withstand sleep deprivation without impairment will develop naturally over time. Efforts to implement fatigue risk management strategies will need to address this assumption if these strategies are to be successfully taken up and effective (Taylor et al. 2019).

Here, the authors highlight their key finding - a problematic assumption held by medical students – and then tell us why that finding matters.

10.4   Making Every Word Count

The Methods piece of your abstract requires you to distill what you did into a couple of sentences, so readers will be able to accurately classify the type of study, the scale and scope of the study, and the approach to data analysis. Remember that this short section also plays a role in establishing your credibility as a researcher. Ensure that your terminology aligns with the methodology you claim, and that it will resonate with experts in the field. Readers may abandon ship if these short sentences don't reassure them that you know what you're doing.

The Results part of the abstract should be meaty and precise. Outline your key results, avoiding terminology that won't be quickly understood. Don't save the good stuff for the paper; results that are critical, novel, or surprising must appear in the abstract. If you have built a significant piece of your Discussion around a particular aspect of your results, highlight that in your abstract.

The Conclusion of the abstract can't just re-state the results. You don't have the space. Instead, use the conclusion to focus on implications. This section is the "so what" of your abstract. What might your results mean for research or for practice in the field? How can your readers use your results? How has the understanding of the problem shifted thanks to your study? Here's the conclusion to the abstract we referenced above – the one that framed the problem as a dilemma:

> This study builds on claims regarding the importance of psychological safety in feedback by clarifying what psychological safety in workplace feedback conversations might look like and identifying associated educator approaches. The results may offer educators practical ways they could work with learners to encourage candid dialogue focused on improving performance (Johnson et al. 2020).

This conclusion speaks directly to the anticipated audience – educators struggling to embed psychological safety in feedback conversations – and offers practical advice they can use. It also offers a promise that reading the paper will be worthwhile, as it will elaborate these ideas in useful ways.

10.5 Final Touches

The finished product should both summarize and persuade. A reader will not only know what your paper is about, but also feel compelled to download, read, and possibly cite it.

Even if your abstract achieves these goals, chances are your first draft will still be longer than allowed. A good abstract is as uncluttered as it is informative. Abstracts call for ruthless editing, and are a great opportunity to sharpen your editorial knife. Find strong verbs that capture the meaning you wish to convey. Chop out non-essential adjectives and adverbs. Avoid duplication. Avoid re-telling the 'what' in the Conclusion, and focus instead on telling the story of why it matters. Check for alignment of the abstract and the paper. The paper should elaborate on ideas highlighted by the abstract; it should not deviate from what the abstract has led readers to expect.

Schimel (2012) outlines three requirements for successful abstracts: simple, concrete, and *unexpected.* Journal reviewers – and reviewers of conference abstracts – always consider a work's originality in deciding its value and its potential to be presented or published. Don't waste the opportunity the abstract offers to highlight what's novel about your work. As a result of reading your abstract, you want readers to feel they have learned something they didn't already know – and perhaps that they would not have expected.

10.6 Conclusion

Great research abstracts are precise, pithy, and persuasive - masterpieces of writing economy. They are the ambassadors of your work. And while a well-written abstract can't compensate for shoddy science, a poorly written abstract can surely bury an excellent study. Give abstracts the time and effort they deserve so that they can effectively champion your work.

See One, Do One, Teach One
1. Try these tasks to engage your skills in concise writing:

   (a) Write an opening sentence for an abstract that captures the problem that your research addresses. Now try a two-sentence opener that allows a bit more nuance. Which do you prefer?
   (b) Write a single sentence that identifies a gap in the literature that your work seeks to address.
   (c) Write a conclusion for your abstract (2 sentences maximum) that highlights the novel contribution your work makes.

2. Pull out an old abstract and practice editing ruthlessly! Can you replace a few verbs with punchier alternatives? Can you declutter by removing unnecessary adjectives and adverbs? Can you ensure that the work's originality shines through?

Now test your powers of persuasion. Share a complete abstract with an honest colleague. Ask them "If you saw this abstract in a conference program, would you want to attend the presentation?" Then ask for a reason for their answer. Yes and no answers can be equally informative!

References

Cook, D. A., & Bordage, G. (2016). Twelve tips on writing abstracts and title: How to get people to use and cite your work. *Medical Teacher, 38*(11), 1100–1104. https://doi.org/10.1080/0142159X.2016.1181732.

Groves, T., & Abbasi, K. (2004). Screening research papers by reading abstracts: Please get the abstract right, because we may use it alone to assess your paper. *BMJ, 329,* 470–471. https://doi.org/10.1136/bmj.329.7464.470.

Johnson, C. E., Keating, J. L., & Molloy, E. K. (2020). Psychological safety in feedback: What does it look like and how can educators work with learners to foster it? *Medical Education, 54*(6), 559–570. https://doi.org/10.1111/medu.14154.

Schimel, J. (2012). *Writing science: How to write papers that get cited, and proposals that get funded.* New York: Oxford University Press USA.

Stupp, R., Mason, W. P., Van Den Bent, M. J., Weller, M., Fisher, B., Taphoorn, M. J., et al. (2005). Radiotherapy plus concomitant and adjuvant Temozolomide for glioblastoma. *New England Journal of Medicine, 352*(10), 987–996. https://doi.org/10.1056/NEJMoa043330.

Taylor, T. S., Raynard, A. L., & Lingard, L. (2019). Perseverance, faith, and stoicism: A qualitative study of medical student perspectives on managing fatigue. *Medical Education, 53*(12), 1221–1229. https://doi.org/10.1111/medu.13998.

Varpio, L., Amiel, J., & Richards, B. F. (2016). Writing competitive research conference abstracts: AMEE Guide No. 108. *Medical Teacher, 38*(9), 863–871. https://doi.org/10.1080/0142159X.2016.1211258.

Venance, S. L., LaDonna, K. A., & Watling, C. J. (2014). Exploring frontline faculty perspectives after a curriculum change. *Medical Education, 48,* 998–1007. https://doi.org/10.1111/medu.12529.

Part II
The Craft

In this book, we approach grammar as tools rather than rules. While most of us can write sentences and paragraphs that are grammatically correct, we may struggle to use the tools of grammar and composition for maximum impact. This section addresses this struggle by offering both basic and advanced tools. Readers may find these chapters most helpful when they already have a solid draft in hand. Don't get bogged down in grammatical refinements when you're trying to put your ideas on the page – that's a recipe for writer's block! Rather, use these chapters selectively to target improvements in particular aspects of a working manuscript draft.

Chapters 11 through 19 focus on basic tools. We've selected some of the most common grammatical struggles that health researchers face, named and explained them, and offered practical solutions. We've also addressed some often-overlooked compositional strategies, including parallel structure, paragraphing, and coherence. Does the world need another book on grammar? Perhaps not. There are, after all, many good resources already available. We've listed a few of our favorites below. But we know that health researchers have neither the time nor the patience to delve into detailed grammar handbooks every time they find themselves stuck with an awkward sentence or a disjointed paragraph. Here, we present nine brief and accessible lessons on grammar and style. Think of them as bite-sized refreshers.

Chapters 20 through 23 focus on advanced tools that can help when your writing just doesn't *sound* right. You have considered the usual suspects - clumsy sentence construction, faulty grammar, unnecessary words – but they are all behaving themselves. Your problem may lie in the more elusive elements of writing: pacing, voice, and modality. These qualities impact how readers think and feel about your subject matter – and about you. You'll know when you've missed the mark when a trusted colleague reviews your work and writes "Watch your tone!" in the margin. Mastering these elements of your writing is tricky, requiring a shift from instinctive to deliberate choices of language and phrasing. In this section, we present tools to help you gain control of pacing, voice, and modality. We've translated lessons from linguistics in order to make them accessible for health researchers. These lessons rarely receive attention in books on scientific writing. Thoughtfully used, they will enhance your versatility as a writer, enable you to more effectively join – or lead -

conversations, and allow you to provoke, challenge, or inspire your readers. On purpose.

A Selection of Grammar Books:

Leech, G. N., Cruickshank, B., & Ivanič, R. (1991). *An A-Z of English grammar and usage*. Walton-on-Thames: Nelson.
O'Conner, P. T. (2010). *Woe is I: the grammarphobe's guide to better English in plain English*. Updated and expanded 3rd ed., 1st Riverhead trade pbk. ed. New York: Riverhead Books.
Pinker, S. (2014). *The sense of style: The thinking person's guide to writing in the 21st century*. New York: Penguin.
Strunk, W., & White, E. B. (2000). *The elements of style* (4th ed.). New York: Longman.
Swan, M. (2016). *Practical English usage* (4th ed.). Oxford: Oxford University Press.
Venolia, J. G. (2001). *Write right! A desktop digest of grammar, punctuation and style* (4th ed.). Berkeley: Ten Speed Press.

Chapter 11
Mastering the Sentence

As writers, we wordsmith tirelessly, chasing the perfect turn of phrase. We experiment with paragraph arrangement, seeking the most logical flow. But, sadly, most of us ignore our sentences. Oh, we look out for sentence fragments and other glaring errors, but we don't think strategically about sentence structure and use it to our advantage. We should. Strong sentences are essential to good writing.

Some sentences stop you in your tracks. You think, 'I wish I'd written that!' When you come across one of these sentences, we encourage you "to take [it] apart, to caress" it (Fish 2011, p. 159). Where does its power come from? As Fish argues, writing great sentences requires more than choosing great words: "Flaubert's famous search for the *mot juste* was not a search for words that glow alone, but for words so precisely placed that in combination with other words, also precisely placed, they carve out a shape in space and time" (p. 2). This chapter aims to refresh some of the basics of sentence structure, so that you, too, can combine words precisely and powerfully.

11.1   Three Types of Sentence

In the English language, there are three types of sentence: simple, compound and complex. A simple sentence is made up of one independent clause, which is a clause that can stand on its own. An independent clause has a <u>subject</u> (a noun or noun phrase representing the main idea) and a **predicate** (a verb or verb phrase representing the main action). Simple does not mean 'short'. Each of the following is a simple sentence:

<u>The professor</u> **goes**.
<u>The professor</u> **goes** reluctantly to the curriculum committee meeting.

© The Author(s), under exclusive license to Springer Nature Switzerland AG 2021
L. Lingard, C. Watling, *Story, Not Study: 30 Brief Lessons to Inspire Health Researchers as Writers*, Innovation and Change in Professional Education 19,
https://doi.org/10.1007/978-3-030-71363-8_11

The professor **goes** reluctantly to the curriculum committee meeting held for the third time this semester.

Wistfully remembering those halcyon days when decisions about teaching were hers alone, the professor **goes** reluctantly to the curriculum committee meeting held for the third time this semester.

A compound sentence is made up of two independent clauses (each with a subject and a **predicate**) that are equal in importance and can each stand alone. The following sentences illustrate how two simple sentences (1a) can be joined by a semi-colon (1b), coordinating conjunction (1c), or a conjunctive adverb (1d):

1a. Reviewer 1 **liked** the paper. Reviewer 2 **loathed** it.
1b. Reviewer 1 **liked** the paper; Reviewer 2 **loathed** it.
1c. Reviewer 1 **liked** the paper, but Reviewer 2 **loathed** it.
1d. Reviewer 1 **liked** the paper; inevitably, Reviewer 2 **loathed** it.

A complex sentence is made up of one independent and one subordinate clause. Each clause has a **predicate**. What distinguishes complex from compound sentences is that, in complex sentences, the two clauses are not equal in importance. The subordinate clause is less important and cannot stand on its own; it is signaled by a *subordinating conjunction* whose function is to join the two clauses.

Although Reviewer 1 **liked** the paper, Reviewer 2 **loathed** it.

In this complex sentence, Reviewer 2's loathing is given more importance than Reviewer 1's liking due to its presence in the independent or main clause.

11.2   The Subject Position

The subject is the noun or noun phrase that the **predicate** refers to, and it is the strongest 'meaning slot' in all three types of sentence. That's where your main idea should be. Imagine that you want to write about the mental health of clinical teachers:

Many factors **can threaten** clinical teachers' sanity, not least among them the hospital's daily inpatient census.

This sentence doesn't highlight teachers' mental health as the main idea. Instead, "factors" has the strongest prominence because it is the subject of the **predicate**. The next version places the main idea in this meaning slot to clearly communicate its importance:

Clinical teachers' sanity **can be threatened** by many factors, not least among them the hospital's daily inpatient census.

Now that you know the power of the subject position slot, don't waste it. Consider the next three examples in which the main idea is intended to be "patient complexity". The first example distracts by making an unimportant word the <u>subject</u> of the **predicate**:

> Studies **suggest** that patient complexity impacts teaching and learning.

The second version weakens the main idea by using a <u>nominalization</u>. This is a noun phrase created from other parts of speech, often a gerund ('ed' or 'ing' verb) or adjective. Nominalizations turn an action into an inanimate object, are usually wordy, and can put the reader into cognitive overload (Casagrande 2010). Consider:

> <u>Complicated patients with multiple problems</u> **impact** teaching and learning.

The third version states the main idea clearly by placing it in the most powerful meaning slot in the sentence, as <u>subject</u> of **the predicate**:

> <u>Patient complexity</u> **impacts** teaching and learning.

An over-complicated subject may also lose impact, even if properly positioned. Consider this mouthful:

> <u>The practice, long valued in apprenticeship models of learning, of ensuring that a teacher has regular opportunities for directly observing the actual performance of a student as they are developing their skills,</u> **reveals** performance deficits that would not have been identified otherwise, informing timely and appropriate educational interventions.

So much ornamentation has been loaded on this subject that the reader is left unsure what the sentence is about. A revision that simplifies the subject heightens the impact:

> <u>Direct observation</u> **reveals** performance deficits that would not have been identified otherwise, informing timely and appropriate educational interventions.

11.3 Using Subject Position Effectively in Complex Sentences

Something interesting happens to the subject position as you change sentence types. A simple sentence has one predicate, and thus offers a single subject position for your main idea:

> <u>Team communication</u> **is** critical.

A compound sentence has two **predicates** and, therefore, two strong <u>subject</u> position slots.

> <u>Team communication</u> **is** critical, but <u>we</u> **don't teach** it.

However, a complex sentence, while it has two **predicates**, has only one strong <u>subject</u> position slot – in the main clause. Therefore, if the sentence's main idea -- "team communication" -- gets placed in the *subordinate clause*, its importance will be diluted:

> *Although team communication is critical*, <u>we</u> **don't teach** it.

The lesson is: don't bury your main idea in the subordinate clause of a complex sentence. It should be the subject of the *main clause*:

> Although we don't teach it, *team communication* is critical.

There are, of course, exceptions, such as when you want to deflect attention from an idea. For instance, when critically summarizing the literature, a diplomatic critique can become inadvertently personalized when the authors are in the main subject position slot:

> Carreras and Larkin argue that reduced duty hours do not improve resident wellness. This claim is not supported by other research in the field.

A complex sentence affords the opportunity to put Carreras and Larkin into the less prominent subject position slot in the *subordinate clause*, while still retaining the substance of the critique:

> While *Carreras and Larkin* argue that reduced duty hours do not improve resident wellness, this claim is not supported by other research in the field.

11.4   Topic Sentences and Paragraph Transitions

A topic sentence is the first sentence in a paragraph, and its role is to signal the main idea that the paragraph will develop. The clearest topic sentences place that main idea in the strongest subject position slot regardless of the sentence type. Topic sentences also serve as transitions to show why one idea/paragraph follows another. Compound and complex sentences make good transition topic sentences. In the compound sentence that follows, for example, the first clause of the sentence summarizes the main idea from the preceding paragraph, while the other clause introduces *the new idea* the current paragraph will develop:

> Competency has received medical educators' attention for over a decade, but *its status as an orthodox religion* is a recent development.

Complex sentences can signpost a transition by placing the topic of the previous paragraph in the subordinate clause and the topic of the new paragraph in the independent clause:

> Although the procedures for carrying out grounded theory research are highly structured, the criteria for evaluating the quality of a grounded theory study are less clear.

Here, the sentence structure helps to turn the spotlight from one idea to the next.

11.5   Conclusion

No sentence type is 'better' than another. Each has its place. Academic writing relies heavily on compound and complex sentences to build arguments by relating ideas. This means that well-placed, simple sentences can be a breath of fresh air and an easy way to highlight a key point. Master sentence structure and subject position and you will find yourself writing clearer, more coherent prose.

See One, Do One, Teach One
1. Scan a draft you are working on for a compound sentence. Try breaking the sentence into two (or more) simple sentences instead. Consider whether this edit strengthens or weakens the writing.
2. Scan that same draft for a complex sentence. Identify the independent clause (the one that can stand alone) and the dependent, or subordinate, clause (the one that can't stand alone). Try swapping the subject position, so that the subject that was in the independent clause moves to the dependent clause and vice versa. What is the impact of this change on your sense of the main idea of the sentence?
3. The next time you are reviewing a colleague's or a student's draft, pay particular attention to transitions. Can you identify a situation where a stronger transition from one paragraph to the next would be beneficial? Instead of merely naming the problem, try your hand at writing a good transition topic sentence, using either a compound or a complex sentence structure.
4. See a sentence that takes your breath away? Something so perfect, so persuasive that you want to quote it? Write it down and try to figure out why it is so effective. Share it with a colleague.

References

Casagrande, J. (2010). *It was the best of sentences, it was the worst of sentences: A writer's guide to crafting killer sentences.* Berkeley: The Speed Press.
Fish, S. (2011). *How to write a sentence and how to read one.* New York: Harper.

Chapter 12
Enlisting the Power of the Verb

Verbs are the engine of a sentence: they propel the prose forward and infuse it with energy. Unfortunately, energy is precisely what much scientific writing lacks. This chapter considers some of the common problems associated with verb use in scientific writing, and offers straightforward solutions that writers can implement to energize their manuscripts.

12.1 Lifeless Default Verbs

One of the main reasons that scientific writing lacks energy is that our 'go-to' verbs are limp and lifeless. Consider this example:

> A recent analysis of social media **shows** that the spread of health misinformation by celebrity figures **is** a growing problem.

This sentence deploys two verbs and each exemplifies a distinct form of lifelessness. The first verb, "shows", is an example of the popularity of "neutral" verbs in scientific writing. Look at your most recent paper: you will undoubtedly find a number of "shows", "suggests", "illustrates", "reports", "describes", "finds", "considers", "presents", "reveals", etc. These verbs are not wrong, but they are boring. Little happens in sentences anchored by them: no stance is taken, no movement occurs, no dramatic tension is introduced. The curious thing is that many writers use such verbs on purpose, because they believe that scientific prose should be dispassionate. This is debatable. Dispassionate scientific prose can have unintended negative effects (Knatterud 2002). Furthermore, it should not be taken as evidence of neutrality or objectivity: as Gross points out, dispassionate prose is "a carefully crafted rhetorical invention", a deliberate attitude of "abstinence" (Gross 1984). Even if a dispassionate voice is your aim, allowing yourself to step outside the narrow range of 'neutral' verbs provides an opportunity for both greater precision and increased energy.

Look at the second verb in the sentence: "is". This ubiquitous little verb – we recommend you use the Find function in your Word document to highlight them all – litters our pages. It is a state-of-being verb, which identifies who or what a noun is, was or will be. In English, most state-of-being verbs are forms of the verb "to be" (am, are, is, was, were, will be, being, been) but other verbs can also function this way, such as "become", "seem" and "appear". State-of-being verbs are necessary, and you cannot rid your prose of them entirely. But you can use them more consciously. Try identifying the ones you need and changing the others to either stative (verbs of thoughts, feelings or sensations) or action verbs (verbs of doing).

The revision below improves on both the neutral verb and the state-of-being verb:

In social media analyses, celebrity figures **contribute** to the growing problem of health misinformation.

Or, you might amp the verb up a bit more:

In social media analyses, celebrity figures **fuel** the growing problem of health misinformation.

If your scientific prose is weakened by default verbs that lack energy, try amping the verb up too far. You can always dial it back as you revise, but it will help you break out of your neutral comfort zone. Keep in mind that the really punchy verbs must be used sparingly: your goal is energy, not melodrama. That said, a single, well-placed verb can capture the reader's attention, as in this lovely example from the opening sentence of a manuscript: "Lack of continuity bedevils the undergraduate clinical teaching environment to the detriment of student learning" (Bates et al. 2013).

Verbs don't work in isolation, so when you revise to punch them up, take note of what happens to the other parts of the sentence. For instance, finding the right verb often makes adverbs unnecessary. Or, alternately, you may retain a weaker verb when you want the reader's attention to land on an adjacent noun or adjective – i.e., when an unusual verb would actually be a distraction. In the sentence "Electronic patient records are labyrinthine", for example, the metaphor of the labyrinth is sufficiently powerful that the tepid state-of-being verb "are" presents a nice counterbalance.

Verbs work closely with their subjects – the noun immediately before the verb – and therefore you should consider how your revisions to verbs affects them. As we discussed in the preceding chapter, the subject of the main verb will attract most of the reader's attention; therefore, you should place central ideas rather than less important ones in that position. In the above sentence, "A recent analysis of social media" featured as the main subject of the main verb. In the revision, this idea has been moved to an opening prepositional phrase and "celebrity figures" now has center stage as the main subject. If you prefer to highlight the idea of "health misinformation", the following revision accomplishes that and still strengthens the verb:

According to social media analyses, health misinformation is increasingly spread by celebrity figures.

One final tip about the relationship between the verb and the subject. Sometimes we force ourselves into using "is" because our subject is a nominalization. This is a noun phrase created from other parts of speech, often a gerund ('ed' or 'ing' verb), and it can put the reader into cognitive overload. The original sentence in this section had one (in bold):

A recent analysis of social media shows that **the spread of health misinformation by celebrity figures** <u>is</u> a growing problem.

Scholarly writing is rife with nominalizations. Helen Sword (2012) calls them "zombie nouns" because they "cannibalize active verbs, suck the lifeblood from adjectives and substitute abstract entities for human beings" (para. 2). We create them by taking other words, like adjectives (precise), verbs (educate) or nouns (patriot) and adding a suffix (ity, tion, or ism) to create a new noun: precision, education, patriotism. Then we like to modify our nominalizations and pile them up:

The **observation** of learners in **clinical placements** is both a **necessity** and a **limitation** in most **medical education programs**.

A chain of nominalizations serves as the subject in this example, requiring the verb "is". The combination is both burdensome and lifeless. To find such nominalizations in your own writing, look at the subject preceding each of the highlighted examples of "is" that your Find function identified. A better verb is usually already in the sentence: in this example, "observe" is a good candidate:

Medical education programs must observe learners, but their ability to do so is limited, particularly in clinical placements.

This example still uses nominalizations (they are difficult to avoid entirely!), but not in a way that demands a limp verb.

12.2 Passive Voice and 'Sounding Scientific'

That little word, "is", and other derivatives of the verb "to be", signal another problem that drains energy from your prose: overuse of the passive voice. Consider this sentence:

False negative test results have been identified as a particular threat to public health and safety.

The passive construction ("have been identified") not only forces the use of the auxiliary verb "to be", but also removes the agent of the action from the sentence. As Richard Lanham (2006) pointed out, you can't tell "who's kicking who?" *(sic)* in a sentence in the passive voice (p. 15). Accordingly, in the example above you can't tell who is doing the "identifying". To identify the passive voice in your sentences, ask yourself "by whom?" If you can't tell, you're dealing with the passive. To revise into active voice, put the agent into the subject position.

There are two ways to convert the above sentence to active; they differ in what they make into the agent of the active verb. The first asks, "identified by whom?" and puts that missing noun into the agent slot, moving "false negative test results" to the objective of the active verb:

> Researchers have identified that false negative test results are a particular threat to public health and safety.

This effectively makes that passive-to-active shift and clearly indicates who is doing the identifying. However, you might not want "researchers" to be the subject of the sentence. You might wish to keep the focus on "False negative test results" while changing the verb to active:

> False negative test results threaten public health and safety.

As this revision illustrates, often there is a strong verb candidate elsewhere in the passive sentence: here, the noun phrase "a particular threat to" becomes the verb "threaten". By giving agency to "false negative test results", this revision keeps that idea in the spotlight.

Traditionally, the passive voice was required in scientific writing because it conveyed objectivity: rigorous methods revealed facts but no person actually created them (Gross 1984). Therefore, many contemporary writers believe that passive voice is a rule they must obey if they want to sound scientific. They are mistaken. In many current scientific genres, active voice is not only allowed, it is preferred. Our point, however, is not that you should avoid passive voice. Rather, we wish you to use it more strategically. In your literature review, for instance, passive voice allows you to be critical of a study, when active voice might come across as an attack on the researchers:

> The question of the patient's role on the healthcare team has been largely overlooked. (passive voice)

> Kershaw et al largely overlook the question of the patient's role on the healthcare team. (active voice)

Similarly, when you want to emphasize the action over the actor, passive voice is preferable:

> University classes across the country were cancelled by officials. (passive)

> Officials cancelled university classes across the country. (active)

If your point is to emphasize the scale of cancellations rather than the officials who made the decision, the passive voice allows you to minimize the decision makers, even to the point of removing the prepositional phrase "by officials".

Rather than blindly implementing active *or* passive voice according to perceived rules, the thoughtful scientific writer uses voice strategically to position herself. For instance, to position on the spectrum of objectivity/subjectivity and achieve nuances of authorial distance, use voice together with narrative point of view. Third person point of view removes the researcher, first person point of view inserts the researcher; passive voice removes the agent, active voice inserts the agent. At least four combinations are possible, illustrated in the following examples from most 'objective' to most 'subjective' sounding:

Existing theories of knowledge translation are challenged by these results. (3rd person, passive voice)

These results challenge existing theories of knowledge translation. (3rd person, active voice, useful if you are writing in a scientific culture that frowns on 1st person point of view)

A challenge to existing theories of knowledge translation is presented by our results. (1st person possessive pronoun "our" with 3rd person subject "results", passive voice)

Our results challenge existing theories of knowledge translation. (1st person possessive pronoun "Our" with 3rd person subject "results", active voice)

We challenge existing theories of knowledge translation with these results. (1st person, active voice: "we" brings the researchers even more into focus than "our results")

Second person point of view is vanishingly rare in empirical scientific writing. However, guidelines and instructional writing sometimes take this perspective. This book, for instance, uses the second person frequently, to reach out and bring you, the reader, into direct conversation with us, the authors. When we use it, we are trying to lessen authorial distance. Guidelines also use the second person but not in a manner that invokes subjectivity. Rather, because guidelines customarily employ verbs in the imperative mood to form commands and requests, they tend to leave the pronoun in ellipsis. With "you" implied but not stated, a greater sense of objectivity is retained, as this excerpt from recent guidelines for remediation in medical education (Chou et al. 2019, p. 325) illustrates:

Do aim to detect a need for remediation early

Do collect relevant data from multiple sources across case content

Do explore multiple causes of learner struggle beyond educational or workplace issues

Even with pronouns in ellipsis, however, the second person point of view lessens authorial distance because it positions the writer as speaking directly to the reader.

12.3   A Note on Verb Tense in the IMRD Format

In a scientific manuscript, conventions exist regarding verb tense. Generally, you should use present tense in the Introduction and the Discussion, and past tense in the Methods and Results. The convention reflects that the study – what you did and what you found – is completed, but the story – the conversation about a problem in the world, and your contribution to that conversation – is current.

There are times, however, when you can't adhere strictly to this convention. For instance, if you wish to present eras of knowledge in your introduction, some of them will need to be in past tense:

> While Georgoff and colleagues reported the first evidence of this phenomenon in 2008, recent research calls into question key aspects of their original description.

We layer tenses like this all the time in our writing, of necessity. Even with such layering, the convention is a useful guideline to keep your tenses from randomly bobbing about.

12.4   Conclusion

In summary, you can improve your writing by identifying your default verbs, selecting active rather than state-of-being verbs, and converting passive to active voice. But the take-home lesson is not that you must purge all passive voice and "to be" verbs from your prose. (The first sentence in this chapter used "to be" as the main verb, and the sky didn't fall.) Rather, the lesson is that such features can produce sluggish academic prose, particularly if you use them pervasively and unconsciously. And, if you are going to revise your verbs, you should consider how they interact with other grammatical features, such as subject position and point of view. Now you are equipped to identify and work on these features, so that your writing takes full advantage of the power of the verb.

See One, Do One, Teach One
1. What are your default verbs? Review your draft and make a list of any verb you use more than twice. Beside each default verb, write at least three alternatives. Keep this list nearby when you're revising.
2. Use the "Find" function to locate all the state of being verbs in your draft: is, are, was, were, being, etc. Assess which you can convert to action verbs. (Don't automatically convert them all; you will need some of them.) When you're converting, keeping amping them up until you're uncomfortable; then dial back just a bit.
3. Find all the passive voice verb constructions in your paper. Identify those that can be changed and convert them to active. (Don't change them all: sometimes you want to emphasize the action, not the actor. Keep those ones in passive voice.) Remember to look elsewhere in the sentence for the best verb candidate – they're likely already in there!
4. Check your tenses.

(continued)

(a) Are the Introduction and Discussion in the present tense?
(b) Are the Methods and Results in the past tense?
(c) Do you have tense drift within sections? If so, address it.

5. Create a personal thesaurus. Start by picking a paper from one of your favorite authors. Flag all the active verbs they use, and then generate a list you can dip into when you need a great verb. Periodically add to your list when you encounter clever verbs in your reading.

References

Bates, J., Konkin, J., Suddards, C., Dobson, S., & Pratt, D. (2013). Student perceptions of assessment and feedback in longitudinal integrated clerkships. *Medical Education, 47*(4), 362–374. https://doi.org/10.1111/medu.12087.

Chou, C. L., Kalet, A., Costa, M. J., Cleland, J., & Winston, K. (2019). Guidelines: The dos, don'ts and don't knows of remediation in medical education. *Perspectives on Medical Education, 8*, 322–338. https://doi.org/10.1007/s40037-019-00544-5.

Gross, A. G. (1984). Style and arrangement in scientific prose: The rules behind the rules. *Journal of Technical Writing and Communication, 14*(3), 241–253. https://doi.org/10.2190/WLJ2-C3LV-PVTH-DYE2.

Knatterud, M. E. (2002). *First do no harm: Empathy and the writing of medical journal articles*. New York: Routledge.

Lanham, R. (2006). *Revising prose* (5th ed.). New York: Pearson Longman.

Sword, H. (2012, July 23). Zombie nouns. *New York Times*. https://opinionator.blogs.nytimes.com/2012/07/23/zombie-nouns/. Accessed 8 Sept 2020.

Chapter 13
The Power of Parallel Structure

Orators have long understood the power of parallel structure. Consider this paragraph from Martin Luther King Jr.'s 2008 "I Have a Dream" speech:

> Now is the time to make real the promises of democracy. Now is the time to rise from the dark and desolate valley of segregation to the sunlit path of racial justice. Now is the time to lift our nation from the quicksands of racial injustice to the solid rock of brotherhood. Now is the time to make justice a reality for all of God's children (King 2008).

This iconic speech stands not only as a masterpiece of oratory, but also as a masterpiece of parallel construction. The paragraph itself is a parallel construction, with its four sentences each leading off with the invocation "Now is the time." And within each of the two middle sentences, evocative contrasts are presented in parallel form.

Audiences – and readers - crave logic and rhythm. Parallel structure delivers both. Using parallel structure effectively is not the sole purview of master orators, however. Once you know where to look for opportunities, you can use parallel structure to enliven your own writing. In this chapter, we will help you to identify and seize opportunities to employ this powerful compositional technique.

13.1 Parallel Structure Defined

Parallel structure simply means that ideas that are similar in content or function are expressed in a similar way (Strunk and White 1999). To present a pair or a series of ideas using parallel structure, each idea should be written in a similar grammatical and stylistic form. Parallel constructions – within sentences or paragraphs – guide readers elegantly through your story. When we use parallel constructions, we *show* our readers how our ideas are linked, rather than forcing them to work to see the connections.

L. Lingard, C. Watling, *Story, Not Study: 30 Brief Lessons to Inspire Health Researchers as Writers*, Innovation and Change in Professional Education 19, https://doi.org/10.1007/978-3-030-71363-8_13

13.2   Parallel Structure in Sentences

Within sentences, there are two key opportunities to use parallel constructions. First, look for situations where you enumerate a series of ideas, and then ensure that each item in the series is similarly constructed. A series might comprise short phrases separated by commas or semicolons, or even set off by numbers. Let's consider an example:

> Faculty members juggled a number of competing responsibilities, including to provide feedback, assessment of learners, and developing curricula.

In this series, the three competing responsibilities are expressed in three different ways: as an infinitive ("to provide"), as a noun ("assessment"), and as a gerund ("developing"). The effect of this eclecticism is that the writing loses momentum, and the reader gets stuck mid-sentence. If each idea were expressed in a similar fashion, the sentence would flow more easily:

> Faculty members juggled a number of competing responsibilities, including **providing feedback, assessing learners, and developing curricula**.

Here each task is expressed as a gerund (an "-ing" verb used as a noun), but there is more than one way to bring parallel structure to this sentence. Each task could also be expressed as a noun:

> Faculty members juggled a number of competing responsibilities, including **feedback provision, learner assessment, and curriculum development**.

The key is to be consistent within a series.

Second, look for opportunities to use joining words to link two ideas within the same sentence. Commonly used joining words include:

Not only. . .but also
Both. . .and
Either. . .or
Neither. . .nor

The trick to making joining words work for you is to ensure that the words that follow the first word or phrase are similar in form to those that follow the second (Pinker 2014):

> Stroke units not only **reduce** mortality, but also **improve** functional outcomes.

In this sentence, the word that follows *not only* ("reduce") is the same form – a present tense verb – as the word that follows *but also* ("improve"), which not only creates a pleasing symmetry, but also reinforces the connection between the two ideas. Fail to maintain consistency across joining words, though, and the magic is lost. A version like this one is sure to trip a reader up:

> Stroke units not only reduce mortality, but also patients' functional outcomes are improved.

Whether joining words are used or not, parallel structure hinges on balance. When ideas are not presented in a symmetrical way, sentences often feel unbalanced, and the impact of linking or contrasting ideas can be diminished. Consider this example:

> While the medical profession values independence and autonomy, the way that we educate medical students tends to be highly structured, with hierarchy playing a prominent role.

The initial dependent clause offers a concise subject ("the medical profession") and highlights two core values, each presented as a single word. The independent clause that follows, though, offers a more complex subject ("the way that we educate medical students") and then elaborates its features in a similarly wordy fashion. The sentence is unbalanced. This revision restores that balance:

> While the **medical profession** values independence and autonomy, **medical schools** tend toward structure and hierarchy.

The subjects are now parallel ("medical profession" and "medical schools"), and the objects of each clause now have a tidy symmetry ("independence and autonomy" versus "structure and hierarchy"). The contrast, as a result, is all the more striking for the reader.

13.3 Parallel Structure in Paragraphs

Just as parallel structure strengthens sentences, so it breathes life into paragraphs. As key building blocks of any manuscript, paragraphs elaborate ideas, advance logic, and build arguments. Consider the following short paragraph about the state of the science on feedback:

> Considerable attention has been paid to the structural aspects of feedback, leading to articles and workshops aimed at educating feedback providers about how to construct and deploy feedback effectively. The issue of learners' responses to feedback has received less attention, although a growing body of literature has been exploring this area. We have not undertaken a critical examination of medicine's learning culture and how it might enable or constrain the exchange of meaningful feedback.

The paragraph is grammatically correct but lacks punch and style. The solution? Create a parallel structure to link the paragraph's three central ideas:

> **We have paid considerable attention** to the structural aspects of feedback, leading to articles and workshops aimed at educating feedback providers about how to construct and deploy feedback effectively. **We have devoted less attention** to learners' responses to feedback, although a growing body of literature has been exploring this area. **And we have virtually ignored** medicine's learning culture and how it might enable or constrain the exchange of meaningful feedback.

Of course, one rarely uses a single writing technique to solve a style problem. Here, we have also used active rather than passive voice constructions for the first two ideas, and we have strengthened the third verb phrase from "we have not undertaken" to "we have virtually ignored."

13.4   Conclusion

As this last example demonstrates, looking for parallel structure – or noticing its absence – can be a powerful editing tool, whether you are working on your own writing or offering feedback on someone else's. The next time you stumble over a sentence or have to reread a paragraph to stitch together its logic, consider whether an injection of parallel structure may be useful. The result will be stronger, clearer, and more persuasive prose.

See One, Do One, Teach One
1. Mundane tasks sometimes offer great opportunities to practice parallel constructions. Find a job description for a position that you hold, and tidy up the list of responsibilities, writing each one using the same grammatical form. Or review the terms of reference for a committee to which you belong, and adjust the list of items that constitute the committee's mandate to ensure parallelism.
2. The next time a colleague asks you to read and give feedback on something they have written, make a point of identifying at least one place where the flow and logic could be improved by parallel structure. Instead of writing "awkward sentence" in the margin, name the problem as a lack of parallel structure, and write a new version that addresses the issue.

References

King, M. L., Jr. (2008). Martin Luther King, Jr.'s "I have a dream" speech: The full text. In P. Finkelman (Ed.), *Milestone documents in American history: Exploring the primary sources that shaped America*. Pasadena: Salem Press. https://online-salempress-com.proxy1.lib.uwo.ca/doi/book//10.3331/mdah.
Pinker, S. (2014). *The sense of style*. New York: Viking.
Strunk, W., & White, E. B. (1999). *The elements of style/by William Strunk, Jr.; with revisions, and introduction, and a chapter on writing by E.B. White* (4th ed.). Boston: Allyn and Bacon.

Chapter 14
Get Control of Your Commas

Please start cutting, Dr. Franklin.
Please start cutting Dr. Franklin.

Comma placement can radically alter the meaning of a sentence. But many of us struggle to know where exactly to put them. How do you decide? Do you treat commas like salt, sprinkling them over your writing according to your personal taste? Have you a vague sense that, like too much salt, too many commas are bad for you? Or are you an adherent of the 'breathing' rule, inserting commas wherever a reader might need an O_2 break? Have you ever wondered why those editing your work have removed one comma but not another?

The purpose of a comma is to separate clauses within a sentence, phrases within a clause or words within a phrase, in order to succinctly and unambiguously express meaning. Seems straightforward, right? Wrong. The comma is arguably the most misunderstood of punctuation tools. Ask someone about comma rules and even those who begin with confidence are likely to trail off apologetically. This is because, although purists feel quite strongly about comma rules and bemoan their misuse in popular punctuation books (Truss 2003), comma use is not fully explained by rules. It depends in part on taste.

As David Crystal (2015) insists in his history of punctuation, variation in comma use is neither infinite nor totally idiosyncratic. It turns out that there are two broad schools of punctuation, and understanding them can help us to unravel the complexities of comma use. In the elocutional school, with its origins in antiquity, commas indicate intonation and pauses in oral speech. In the grammatical school, which arose with the advent of the printing press, commas express grammatical relations among parts of the sentence. What's tricky is that both approaches are still alive and well, so that most of us have been trained, explicitly or implicitly, to use a bit of both in our writing.

The original version of this chapter was revised: Epigraph was corrected. The correction to this chapter is available at https://doi.org/10.1007/978-3-030-71363-8_31

© The Author(s), under exclusive license to Springer Nature Switzerland AG 2021, corrected publication 2021
L. Lingard, C. Watling, *Story, Not Study: 30 Brief Lessons to Inspire Health Researchers as Writers*, Innovation and Change in Professional Education 19, https://doi.org/10.1007/978-3-030-71363-8_14

Getting control of your commas requires distinguishing between rules and preferences, which map closely onto the grammatical and elocutional schools of comma use. The aim of this chapter is to help you ascertain when commas are prohibited, when they are necessary, and when they are unnecessary but acceptable as a matter of preference.

14.1   Comma Rules

This list is not exhaustive, nor is it in any particular order of priority. Based on our experience reviewing and mentoring the scholarly writing of health researchers, these are among the most common comma errors.

When the **subject** and its <u>verb</u> are side by side, never separate them with a comma.

> *Incorrect*: **Pediatric inpatients between the ages of ten and fifteen,** <u>participated</u> in the study.
> *Correct*: **Pediatric inpatients between the ages of ten and fifteen** <u>participated</u> in the study.

If you are inclined to place a comma between your subject and verb, this usually signals that your subject is too long and the sentence should be reworked to shorten it. Inserting an elocutionary comma in this case – a comma that creates a pause so the reader can absorb the long subject and note the coming verb – is incorrect.

When a list follows a <u>verb</u>, there should not be a comma separating the verb from the list:

> *Incorrect*: The factors influencing physicians' decisions about formal research training <u>are</u>, debt, role models, program culture and personal ambition.
> *Correct*: The factors influencing physicians' decisions about formal research training <u>are</u> debt, role models, program culture and personal ambition.

Commas are not used on their own to join independent sentences:

> *Incorrect*: I came to medical school, I saw all the work I had to do, incredibly I conquered it.
> *Correct*: *I came to medical school. I saw all the work I had to do. Incredibly, I conquered it.*

In a compound sentence, a comma is necessary before the **conjunction** that joins the two independent clauses:

> *Incorrect*: Frontline nurses agreed to participate in the new assessment scheme **but** they were not enthusiastic about its chances of success.
> *Correct*: Frontline nurses agreed to participate in the new assessment scheme, **but** they were not enthusiastic about its chances of success.

In compound sentences that use a **conjunctive adverb**, a semi-colon should precede the adverb and a comma follow it:

> *Incorrect*: Frontline nurses agreed to participate in the new assessment, **however** they were not enthusiastic about its chances of success.
> *Incorrect*: Frontline nurses agreed to participate in the new assessment, **however,** they were not enthusiastic about its chances of success.

Correct: Frontline nurses agreed to participate in the new assessment; **however**, they were not enthusiastic about its chances of success.

A comma is necessary between the main clause and subordinate clause in a complex sentence, regardless of which clause comes first:

Incorrect: Although the new electronic patient record is not believed to influence medical teaching there has been no systematic study of its educational effects.

Correct: Although the new electronic patient record is not believed to influence medical teaching, there has been no systematic study of its educational effects.

Correct: There has been no systematic study of the new electronic patient record's educational effects, although it is not believed to influence medical teaching.

With relative clauses, a comma signals that the detail is parenthetical, while no comma indicates that the detail is necessary to the meaning of the sentence.

Parenthetical: The faculty, who had been carefully trained, were expert clinical teachers.

Necessary: The faculty who had been carefully trained were expert clinical teachers.

In the parenthetical version, all faculty had been carefully trained and all were expert teachers. You can imagine replacing the commas with brackets in this version. In the necessary, or 'restrictive relative', version, only the faculty who had been carefully trained were expert clinical teachers; the implication is that other faculty who were not carefully trained were not expert clinical teachers,

14.2 Comma Preferences

Editorial preferences for comma use abound, and they have evolved across history, with a more modern, minimalist approach to commas prevailing now in comparison with a hundred years ago (Crystal 2015). Complicating matters, comma preferences are often presented as if they were rules. These commas, however, are not obligatory. In deciding whether to use them, you will usually be weighing their effect on elocution: do they help the reading process? According to Crystal (2015), two factors are important in such decisions: (1) the length of the phrase to be separated and (2) the tightness of its semantic link with the rest of the sentence. The longer the length, the more likely the comma. The tighter the semantic link, the less likely the comma. The trouble is that sometimes these two factors are in tension, but that is beyond the scope of this chapter.

Commas can be used, or not, to set off 'wind-ups' (Lanham 2006), those introductory phrases at the head of the sentence:

In this qualitative research study, the focus was residents' experiences of workplace-based assessment.

In this qualitative research study the focus was residents' experiences of workplace-based assessment.

In this qualitative research study conducted by Sinclair et al during the shift to competency-based medical education in Canada, the focus was residents' experience of workplace-based assessment.

The last, longer wind-up is much easier to read with an elocutionary comma separating it from the main clause, and some would argue that this comma is grammatically obligatory. As a general rule, phrases longer than 7 words are more likely to take a comma in such cases (Crystal 2015).

Another matter of preference is whether there should be a comma before the conjunction joining the last two items in a list – called the 'serial' or Oxford comma:

> The committees requiring new members include occupational safety, finance, promotion and tenure, and strategic planning.

Newspaper articles rarely use this comma; academic writing often does, but it varies by publishing press. When in doubt, check the usage for the journal you are writing for. And be consistent: whatever you choose, make it the same throughout the manuscript.

If you find yourself inserting many elocutionary commas to create pauses and ease reading in a sentence, this is likely a signal that your sentence is too long:

> Before embracing subjectivity, increasingly recognized as a key dimension of rater cognition, the medical education community needs to consider how subjectivity and objectivity interact and, even more critically, how current assessment instruments are structured to prompt, or inhibit, particular rater responses.

This sentence breaks none of the comma rules outlined above. In total, however, this pile of commas signals a sentence that is overly complex and meandering. Consider breaking up such cumbersome constructions into a series of shorter, clearer sentences. This version is better:

> Subjectivity is increasingly recognized as a key dimension of rater cognition. Before the medical education community embraces subjectivity, however, it should consider how subjectivity and objectivity interact. Even more critically, it should consider how current assessment instruments prompt or inhibit particular rater responses.

14.3   Conclusion

Comma use can be baffling. If you know the basic comma rules and the logic that governs comma preferences, you can better decide when a comma is prohibited, necessary, or a matter of personal taste. Consistency in these decisions is critical to ensuring clarity in your writing.

See One, Do One, Teach One
1. Print out a page of your writing. Circle all the commas. For each comma you found, consider the seven comma rules outlined in this chapter – are you breaking any?
2. Review your writing and identify the longest sentences. Often, the commas in such sentences could be changed to help the reader keep track of the

(continued)

meaning. Consider whether you might change any of the commas to a stronger punctuation point such as a semi-colon or period.
3. Can't find many commas in your writing? Ask someone else to review a paragraph you've written and suggest whether it needed commas for clarity as they read.

References

Crystal, D. (2015). *Making a point: The persnickety story of English punctuation*. New York: St. Martin's Press.
Lanham, R. (2006). *Revising prose* (5th ed.). New York: Pearson Longham.
Truss, L. (2003). *Eats, shoots & leaves: The zero tolerance approach to punctuation*. London: Profile Books.

Chapter 15
Avoiding Prepositional Pile-Up

What's wrong with the following sentence?

> After receiving research ethics approval from the review boards at three teaching hospitals affiliated with two universities in urban Ontario, Canada, we asked clinical and educational leaders in each hospital to identify inter-professional clinical health care teams with reputations for strong collaborations and managerial/administrative support.

This sentence is long, but there's no golden rule about sentence length. It's complex, but it doesn't commit any grammatical errors. Its main clause is well-formed, with a clear subject (we) and an active main verb (asked). It's properly punctuated. Then why is it so hard to digest?

Diagnosis: prepositional pile-up. This sentence – one of our own (Lingard et al. 2012, p. 1763) – features nine prepositions:

> **After** receiving research ethics approval **from** the review boards **at** three teaching hospitals affiliated **with** two universities **in** urban Ontario, Canada, <u>we asked clinical and educational leaders</u> **in** each hospital **to** identify inter-professional <u>clinical health care teams</u> **with** reputations **for** strong collaborations and managerial/administrative support.

These prepositions require the reader to sift through a host of details that elaborate the main clause – 'we asked clinical and educational leaders'. Prepositional pile-up like this creates cognitive burden for the reader, making it difficult for her to see through the details to the essence of a sentence. This chapter will help you to identify prepositions, diagnose the extent to which your writing contains prepositional pile-up, and edit to address this problem when you find it.

© The Author(s), under exclusive license to Springer Nature Switzerland AG 2021   101
L. Lingard, C. Watling, *Story, Not Study: 30 Brief Lessons to Inspire Health Researchers as Writers*, Innovation and Change in Professional Education 19,
https://doi.org/10.1007/978-3-030-71363-8_15

15.1   What's a Preposition?

The most common prepositions are the "little words": in, to, with, on, at, of, for. Prepositions show relationships of: direction (e.g., from, to), place (e.g., under, over, in), time (e.g., before, after, during, until), cause (e.g., by, of, in order that), manner (e.g., with, among, against) and amount (e.g., most of, both of). Prepositions sit at the beginning of 'prepositional phrases' which include the preposition's <u>object</u>: on <u>the test</u>; from <u>the review board</u>; with <u>two universities</u>; in <u>urban Ontario, Canada</u>.

Prepositional phrases serve an important function, allowing the writer to provide additional detail about the main action. But a writer must ask herself, are these additional details really necessary? And when they pile up into strings of multiple prepositional phrases, can the reader sort through them without getting overwhelmed?

15.2   What's the Problem?

In the sentence above, a string of five prepositional phrases provides additional detail about the main action before the reader encounters that main action:

> **After** receiving research ethics approval – *Ethics approval from where?* – **from** the review boards – *Which review boards?* – **at** three teaching hospitals – *Which hospitals?* – affiliated **with** two universities – *Where were these universities?* – **in** urban Ontario, Canada, <u>we asked clinical and educational leaders</u> . . .

Such strings of prepositional phrases zoom in closer and closer on detail. But because they accumulate before the main clause, they can distract the reader from the central thrust of the sentence.

As Pinker (2014) explains, "The human mind can only do a few things at a time, and the order in which information comes in affects how that information is handled" (p. 83). According to this logic, prepositional pile-up early in a sentence risks overwhelming the reader. It can do so, for instance, by creating a long noun phrase in the subject position (underlined), which directly precedes the main verb "is". The following is an example:

> <u>The attempt **to** articulate milestones relevant **to** both specific activities **of** practice and stages **of** trainee development</u> is **at** the center **of** our current competency-based assessment activities.

As this example illustrates, long noun phrases in the subject position are often followed by a form of the verb 'to be'. As discussed in Chap. 12, the verb 'to be' is a flag for limp writing, and it is worth analyzing your drafts to see how you're using it.

15.3   What's the Solution?

The following revision addresses both the prepositional pile-up and the weak verb:

> Competency-based assessment requires the articulation **of** milestones reflecting both specific practice activities and training stages.

The revision reduces the number of prepositional phrases, partly by converting phrases like 'stages **of** trainee development' to 'training stages'. But it also moves the main subject and verb – 'Competency-based assessment requires' – to earlier in the sentence, so that the reader is anchored by the main action before encountering layers of detail.

We're not advocating that you purge the detail from your writing. But where you do choose to elaborate the detail through layers of prepositional phrases, remember Pinker's point about the order of information. Place details after an early and simple subject-verb-object construction, so that the reader has a mental folder to house them:

> We engaged an advisory panel **of** digital health knowledge users **to** provide input **at** strategic stages **of** the scoping review **to** enhance the relevance **of** findings and inform dissemination activities (Soobiah et al. 2020).

This example has six prepositional phrases but it's not overwhelming for the reader. The subject-verb-object comes first and everything that follows is just more detail about the "advisory panel". To appreciate the advantage of putting the subject-verb-object early to 'open the folder' in the reader's brain so that they have a place to file the details, try flipping the sentence:

> **To** provide input **at** strategic stages **of** the scoping review **to** enhance the relevance **of** findings and inform dissemination activities, we engaged an advisory panel **of** digital health knowledge users.

In this version, the reader must wade through five prepositional phrases *before* coming to the subject-verb-object, accumulating details with nowhere to put them.

Fixing prepositional pile-up is not simply a matter of purging prepositions from your writing. Prepositions are necessary, and we rarely craft a sentence without them. (In this chapter, for instance, only a handful of sentences are preposition-free.) When revising, you need to identify prepositions that can be removed without changing meaning (stage **of** trainee development → training stage) and ascertain whether the placement of prepositions in your sentences is taxing the reader's attention.

Sometimes, the best solution to prepositional pile-up is to break the sentence into two. Our first example requires this revision technique:

> We received research ethics approval **from** three urban teaching hospitals **in** Ontario, Canada. Clinical and educational leaders were asked **to** identify inter-professional healthcare teams reputed **to** be collaborative and administratively well-supported.

Other times, reordering the sentence to put the subject-verb before the prepositional phrases is the fix you need. And sometimes, you need to ask yourself if all those details are truly necessary for the reader. You may like them, but what do they really add? The next two examples, a draft and published version of a sentence in one of our papers, illustrate this solution:

> Our tacit acceptance **of** the illusion **of** supervision – made possible when we use fluent telling **as** a proxy **for** competent doing and thinking **in** exchanges **between** supervisors and trainees – is necessary to maintain our sense **of** the safety **of** this clinical training system **in** healthcare.

> Our tacit acceptance of the illusion of supervision – made possible when we use fluent telling as a proxy for competent doing and thinking – is necessary to maintain this clinical training system (Lingard and Goldszmidt 2020, p. 180).

The second, published version has removed five prepositional phrases that we judged less necessary. It is more readable than the first. Honestly, though, if we had it to do over, we would anchor the sentence with an earlier and simpler subject-verb-object and break it into two:

> We tacitly accept the illusion of supervision when we use fluent telling as a proxy for competent doing and thinking. This tacit acceptance is necessary to maintain our sense of the safety of this clinical training system.

Now, isn't that better?

15.4 Conclusion

Prepositions like to pile up in academic writing. This might be because, in order to meet journal word-length requirements, writers try to cram as much detail into as few words as possible. (It's no accident that our first example comes from a methods section; we were probably trying to detail the nuances of the study sample efficiently.) Preposition-heavy writing may give writers a false sense that they are using words efficiently, when in fact they are both adding to the word count and creating verbal quicksand for the reader. Now that you know what prepositional pile-up looks like and how it affects readers, you can lighten the prepositional load in your writing.

See One, Do One, Teach One
1. Choose a few paragraphs from your writing and circle all the prepositions. Underline the prepositional phrases that they introduce. When you find phrase strings (many prepositional phrases in a row), highlight those in yellow. Now, step back and look for patterns:

   (a) Do you use a lot of strings, or not?
   (b) Where in the sentence do your prepositional phrases come? Before the main action (the subject-verb-object) or after?

(continued)

2. Revise a sentence that has prepositional pile-up.

   (a) Try to remove as many prepositions as you can.
   (b) For those that remain, see if you can rewrite the sentence so that the details of the prepositional phrases follow the main subject and verb.

References

Lingard, L., & Goldszmidt, M. (2020). The rhetorical possibilities of a multi-metaphorical view of clinical supervision. In A. Bleakley (Ed.), *Routledge handbook of the medical humanities* (pp. 176–184). New York: Routledge.

Lingard, L., Vanstone, M., Durrant, M., Fleming-Carroll, B., Lowe, M., Rashotte, J., Sinclair, L., & Tallett, S. (2012). Conflicting messages: Examining the dynamics of leadership on interprofessional teams. *Academic Medicine, 87*(12), 1762–1767. https://doi.org/10.1097/ACM.0b013e318271fc82.

Pinker, S. (2014). *The sense of style: The thinking person's guide to writing in the 21st century!* New York: Penguin.

Soobiah, C., Cooper, M., Kishimoto, V., Bhatia, R. S., Scott, T., Maloney, S., et al. (2020). Identifying optimal frameworks to implement or evaluate digital health interventions: A scoping review protocol. *BMJ Open, 10*, e037643. https://doi.org/10.1136/bmjopen-2020-037643.

Chapter 16
Avoiding Clutter:
Using Adjectives and Adverbs Wisely

When you catch an adjective, kill it.

– Mark Twain

We recently happened on a study that quantified adjective and adverb use in a huge corpus of scientific literature. The author found that researchers in the social sciences and humanities used a lot more adverbs (but marginally fewer adjectives) than researchers in the natural and applied sciences (Lei 2016). As qualitative social scientists, we barely stifled yawns. But one finding leapt off the page. For comparison, the author also quantified the adjectives and adverbs in Mark Twain's *Huckleberry Finn.* Twain was much more sparing with adjectives, using them at less than half the frequency of scientific writers (although he was rather more promiscuous with adverbs). Yet while scientific writing suffers from chronic dullness, Twain's writing epitomizes evocative storytelling. The author of this study concluded that researchers – especially social scientists – needed to heed Twain's advice to rein in their use of modifiers. But perhaps there's more to it than that.

It's easy to pick on modifiers. Adjectives and adverbs are derided as clutter in scientific writing, and writers are urged to expunge them. But the right approach isn't so draconian. Adjectives and adverbs are linguistic tools. Just because some writers have misused tools doesn't mean all writers should avoid them. The sparing and selective use of modifiers will perk up your writing just as surely as their excessive use will bog it down. But how to find that balance?

16.1 Intent

Let's start with a reminder of the purpose that modifiers serve. Adjectives modify nouns, making them more distinctive. A strong adjective is not only precise, but also necessary to the meaning of a sentence. When we speak of "informed" consent, "end-of-life" decisions, and "statistical" significance, we conjure specific meanings for readers – interpretations not contained within the nouns themselves. Adjectives

L. Lingard, C. Watling, *Story, Not Study: 30 Brief Lessons to Inspire Health Researchers as Writers*, Innovation and Change in Professional Education 19, https://doi.org/10.1007/978-3-030-71363-8_16

in scientific writing also draw comparisons; we use them to show when a treatment is *more effective* than placebo or when a drug is *riskier* than anticipated. Sound scientific writing depends on such adjectives.

Adverbs modify verbs, adjectives, or other adverbs. They express manner (how?), time (when?), place (where?), and degree (how much?) (Hale 2013, p. 96). Like adjectives, their use should be restricted to situations where they add new information rather than duplicating or over-adorning existing information. Adverbs should *usefully* change the words they modify; otherwise, they become distractions.

Adjectives and adverbs may help to persuade by intensifying the impact of the words they modify. Consider the following excerpt from the opening paragraph of a study of medical errors (adjectives in italics, adverbs in bold):

> **However**, isolating the factors underlying *specific* types of errors has proved to be a *formidable* task. The types of errors that occur vary **widely** because of the *extreme* complexity and heterogeneity of the tasks involved in *medical* care. **Furthermore**, many of the **most** *devastating* errors happen **too infrequently** for *observational* or *single-institution* studies to identify the risk factors and patterns of causation (Gawande et al. 2003, p. 229).

Adjectives like "formidable" and "devastating" grab the reader's attention; the use of the adverb "most" amps up the tension. This strategy pre-empts the reader asking "so what?" about the relevance of the research. But this strategy is also best used in moderation, lest readers tire of the arm-waving.

This passage also illustrates the fondness that scientific writers have for a special type of adverb: the conjunctive adverb. Hale describes these words as "hybrids that share the DNA of both adverbs and conjunctions" (Hale 2013, p. 97). Conjunctive adverbs allow writers to link ideas; used effectively, they improve the logic and flow of writing, guiding readers through complex arguments. But while a well-placed "however" can signal that a counterargument is coming, a paper littered with "howevers", "moreovers" and "furthermores" can try a reader's patience. As with most special grammatical tools, the key here is judicious and purposeful use. Also remember: conjunctive adverbs are not interchangeable. We all have our favorites, but we must guard against using them indiscriminately. If we send in a "however" to do the work of a "furthermore", we confuse readers by raising their expectations for a counterargument, then instead offering an elaboration.

Modifiers offer something else to scientific writers. They signal uncertainty or insecurity, and sometimes that's exactly what scientific writers need to express. Adjectives like "tentative" or "preliminary" and adverbs like "probably" and "generally" allow us to hedge. And hedging, as we show in Chaps. 21 and 22, can allow us to politely enter conversations without alienating readers and peers.

16.2 Hazards

Less is more. Scientific writers can overuse modifiers, gumming up their prose. Writers should pause to consider whether they need to refer to "clear" evidence or to give "serious" consideration. And if they decide that a modifier is called for, one good one generally trumps two or more. Strings of adjectives describing the same noun tend to dilute rather than heighten impact. Describing feedback as an "indispensable" element of clinical learning might strengthen your case; saying that feedback is "essential and indispensable" begins to weaken it. If you do opt for a series of adjectives, each word must contribute distinct nuance. If you find yourself writing the phrase 'high-stakes summative' assessment, for example, ask yourself whether both "high-stakes" and "summative" are required. You might conclude that there is some redundancy, as high-stakes assessments are almost always summative. On the other hand, writing about a 'high-stakes workplace-based' assessment tells the reader two different things about the assessment – extra nuance that justifies both adjectives.

Redundant modifiers weaken prose, even when they are compelling words in their own right. While intended to enhance the meaning of a verb, noun or adjective, they can instead compete with it, sapping the sentence of its intended impact. Describing a health care system as "labyrinthine" has more power than calling it "bafflingly labyrinthine", for example.

Using adverbs to intensify adjectives is dicey in scientific writing. Pinker notes that "unmodified adjectives and nouns tend to be interpreted categorically: honest means 'completely honest.' As soon as you add an intensifier, you're turning an all-or-none dichotomy into a graduated scale" (Pinker 2014, p. 45) For example, the adjective "significant" often has a categorical meaning, signaling that a p-value bar has been met. The intensified "highly significant" gilds the lily, and may make the reader say, "I'll be the judge of that, thank you." Efforts to intensify may instead undermine; as we showed above, a little arm-waving can grab a reader's attention, but too much can raise suspicions that our arguments are more tenuous than we'd like to admit.

The cardinal adverbial sin is to use an adverb to prop up a weak verb or adjective. In these cases, the problem lies not with the modifier, but with the word that relies on it. Earlier in this chapter, we suggested that adverbs should "usefully" change the meaning of the words they modify. We might have instead said that adverbs should "refine" or "focus" the meaning of the words they modify; these stronger verbs render the adverb "usefully" unnecessary.

Finally, beware of adjectives or adverbs that describe the reactions of the observer as opposed to the qualities of the thing being observed (Hale 2013, p. 92). Adjectives like "interesting", "important", and "surprising" – and their adverbial cousins "interestingly", "importantly", and "surprisingly" – love to worm their way into scientific writing. Sometimes, we even combine them for effect; we have all been tempted to write double modifiers like "particularly interesting" or "especially noteworthy".

Don't give in. As C. S. Lewis noted, "Let me taste for myself, and you'll have no need to tell me how I should react to the flavour" (Lewis 1960, p. 318).

16.3   Scaffolding

Adjectives and adverbs create the scaffolding on which we build our drafts. They can be as essential as caffeine and deadlines. Writing about modifiers, Hale cautions against "authorial laziness", that habit of piling on "the first flabby words that come to mind" (Hale 2013, p. 101). But tasking modifiers with maintaining the momentum of drafting is not lazy. Drafting and editing are different activities. When editing, adverbs (and, to a lesser extent, adjectives) act as signal flares. They point to places in our writing where we need to tighten the screws – to search for stronger verbs, sharper adjectives, or more distinctive nouns. But when drafting, such searches become rabbit holes, creating unwelcome and time-consuming distractions from just getting the draft done.

It's okay if you use modifiers early in your writing process, when you're shaping the story. Once the story has been tidied up, the scaffolding can come down. Just because words are edited out of the final product doesn't mean they weren't essential drivers of the process.

16.4   Art

While we opened this chapter with a quote from Mark Twain, the quote was incomplete, and didn't capture the essence of his advice. He went on to clarify: "When you catch an adjective, kill it. No, I don't mean utterly, but kill most of them--then the rest will be valuable." This is the art of using modifiers. Pick your spots.

Songwriters are masters of the short form, expressing complex thoughts in punchy phrases. But even they recognize that a well-placed adverb or two can sometimes work magic. In Dolly Parton's iconic song "Jolene", she uses evocative imagery but is sparing with adverbs, until she unleashes two in the same sentence:

I can easily understand
How you could easily take my man

Remarkably, she uses the *same* adverb twice, flouting the rules of good writing construction. But the adverb is spot-on (both times), conveying just the right mix of surrender and desperation that the song requires. It's hard to imagine that any wordsmithing would have improved this line.

16.5 Conclusion

The lesson? While modifiers can clutter our prose, eradicating them may rob it of impact. Like a good songwriter, a savvy writer knows just when to leave one or two well-placed modifiers for maximum effect. The trick is to choose wisely.

See One, Do One, Teach One
1. Select a paragraph from a draft you're working on (or, if you're feeling courageous, from a paper you've already published). Highlight all the adjectives in the paragraph. Then chop out half of those adjectives. How did you decide which ones made the cut?
2. Take a section of a draft and highlight all the adverbs you can find. Subject each to the modifier test: does the adverb adjust or fine-tune the meaning of the word it modifies? See how many adverb/verb pairs you can replace with a stronger verb that has the same meaning.
3. When offering feedback on a student's or a colleague's draft, look for modifiers that tell you how you as a reader should feel. How do you react to these words? Flag examples where they are unnecessary or even irritating, and explain why in your feedback.

References

Gawande, A. A., Studdert, D. M., Orav, E. J., Brennan, T. A., & Zinner, M. J. (2003). Risk factors for retained instruments and sponges after surgery. *New England Journal of Medicine, 348*, 229–235. https://doi.org/10.1056/NEJMsa021721.

Hale, C. (2013). *Sin and syntax: How to craft wicked good prose.* New York: Three Rivers Press.

Lei, L. (2016). When science meets cluttered writing: Adjectives and adverbs in academia revisited. *Scientometrics, 107*, 1361–1372. https://doi.org/10.1007/s11192-016-1896-3.

Lewis, C. S. (1960). *Studies in words.* London: Cambridge University Press.

Pinker, S. (2014). *The sense of style.* New York: Viking.

Chapter 17
From Semi-Conscious to Strategic Paragraphing

All writing is a march of paragraphs, each of which provides
a clear step forward in the progress of the piece.
–Charles Euchner

Deep in the writer's subcortex lives the primitive instinct to paragraph. We tap away at our laptop keyboards, periodically hitting the ↵ key to send the cursor back to the left margin. Often this act is only semi-conscious: when our writing session ends, we are as surprised to find our work paragraphed as we are to find our coffee mug empty. Other times, we paragraph visually, hitting ↵ because the paragraph looks too long, or because we want to change topics and we know that white space is the way to signal this on the page. Such semi-conscious paragraphing isn't necessarily *wrong*, but it is problematic. Paragraphs are not just a structural feature of writing, they are a rhetorical device, arguably the most powerful tool we have for organizing and developing an argument. Not paying them careful attention, therefore, limits the persuasiveness and clarity of our writing. This chapter introduces a language for thinking strategically about paragraphing and addressing common pitfalls.

17.1   What Is a Paragraph?

A paragraph is a single unit of thought made up of a group of related sentences. Two principles govern effective paragraphing: unity and coherence. Unity refers to the paragraph's single main idea, which should be readily identifiable, introduced up front, developed convincingly, and concluded. Coherence refers to the relationships among the sentences in the paragraph. Each sentence should participate in the main idea and be arranged to create the sense of a developing logic rather than a random list. Think of your paragraphs as a sort of "macropunctuation" (Reeves and Leventhal 2012, p. 298), sending messages to the reader to ease reading and support understanding.

© The Author(s), under exclusive license to Springer Nature Switzerland AG 2021   113
L. Lingard, C. Watling, *Story, Not Study: 30 Brief Lessons to Inspire Health
Researchers as Writers*, Innovation and Change in Professional Education 19,
https://doi.org/10.1007/978-3-030-71363-8_17

Many health researchers struggle to write because of situational issues. *They write in time increments of minutes, not hours or days. They lack a quiet workspace conducive to sustained focus. They work in isolation, without access to a group of writers to provide feedback. And they inhabit an institutional culture that may prevent the vulnerability necessary to even ask for such feedback.* **According to Sword (2017), such situational factors can be as detrimental to writing productivity as more technical challenges such as grammar or writing in a second language.** <u>Given this, situational issues should be addressed in faculty development programs directed at health professional writers.</u>

Fig. 17.1 Illustration of the Dunleavy paragraph model

A popular model for achieving paragraph unity and coherence in academic writing is the Topic/Body/Tokens/Wrap structure (Dunleavy 2003). The first sentence of a paragraph is the Topic sentence; it announces the paragraph's main idea. *Body sentences* develop that core idea. **Token sentences** are woven through the Body, providing illustrative examples or supporting evidence. The <u>Wrap</u> sentence pulls the paragraph argument together and also often provides a link forward to the next paragraph. Figure 17.1 illustrates this model:

The Topic/Body/Tokens/Wrap structure provides a vocabulary for paying careful attention to paragraphs – your own, or those of the writers you're supporting. Critical questions we can now ask include:

- Does the first sentence clearly signal the Topic of the paragraph? In the example above, the use of a simple sentence structure (subject, verb, object) helps to ensure that the reader can't miss the main idea (see Chap. 11). In paragraphs that develop sophisticated ideas, simple sentences for the Topic and the Wrap can improve clarity.
- Do the Body sentences all develop the main idea, or are some a distraction? Is there a logical pattern to their organization? Pattern is a rhetorical strategy that makes a paragraph more convincing. In the example above, the organizing pattern is one of broadening scope, from the writer's time and space to their peer group and their institution. Parallel structure (see Chap. 13) is also used to cluster the body sentences elaborating situational issues: "They write…They lack…They work…And they inhabit…".
- Are the Token sentences placed strategically? Not all paragraphs have Token sentences, because not all Body sentences require a Token. In the example above, for instance, there are four Body sentences followed by one supporting Token sentence. There is no rule about the number or positioning of Tokens; however, Dunleavy (2003) warns that they are digressive by nature and therefore require careful signposting to maintain coherence, particularly when a series of Tokens is used. They may also be a good site for editing when you wish to tighten the argument: ask yourself if all your Tokens are necessary, and delete those that are superfluous or tangential.
- Is there a Wrap sentence? Many paragraphs simply end, without concluding. A good Wrap sentence should not just repeat the Topic sentence, or the paragraph

risks feeling that it has not developed meaningfully. In the example above, the Wrap introduces the implications of situational writing issues for faculty development, thus pointing forward to the next paragraph which will elaborate relevant faculty development approaches. Wrap sentences can also be written to elaborate a Topic that was introduced simply. Think of the Wrap sentence as the writer's opportunity to move their argument along: this last sentence doesn't restate the points made in the paragraph, it summarizes with an eye to the overarching story being crafted. Using the Wrap sentence in this way can help to ensure that, in hindsight, the reader understands the paragraph as *developing* an argument rather than meandering through some points.

17.2 Paragraphing Pitfalls

Paragraphing is a challenging skill to develop. Let's consider some of the ways writers can get off track, and how these problems can be addressed.

17.2.1 The Infinity Paragraph

Some paragraphs go on forever, straining the reader's cognitive resources. This strain signals two problems. The first is a problem of internal coherence: i.e., the transitions between sentences within a paragraph that show relationships among them and create a sense of unity. The second is a problem of external coherence: i.e., the connections between this paragraph and the paragraphs that came before it in the paper's unfolding argument. Readers not only get lost inside the infinity paragraph; they forget how they got to it in the first place. There is no rule to follow to decide if your paragraph has gotten too long: the length of a paragraph is determined by the demands of content, not by the space on the page. Generally, though, if your paragraph is more than a manuscript page in length, or about 250 words, ask yourself if it can be broken into two or three paragraphs. Crafted properly, with strong transitions between them to support external coherence, three shorter paragraphs may help you to develop your argument in a more persuasive manner.

17.2.2 The Hiccup Paragraph

This paragraph ends as abruptly as it started, leaving the reader uncertain how – or if – the argument has developed. British grammarian H.W. Fowler (1926) defined the paragraph as a unit of thought rather than length, and made the point that a sequence of short paragraphs is as irritating as long ones are tiring. So what qualifies as too short? Dunleavy (2014) suggests that paragraphs of fewer than 100 words should be targeted for development. A very short paragraph can be used to provide emphasis in an argument, but a series of them could be a sign that your ideas are not well-developed. You can think of your paragraphs as links in a chain: the strength of each link is dependent on how well that paragraph develops its idea. If you tend toward hiccup paragraphs, one way to improve is to see if a sequence of them can be combined. Combining them will force you to articulate the relationships among these ideas, which is part of the work of developing an idea rather than simply stating it.

17.2.3 The Blindfold Paragraph

A blindfold paragraph leaves the reader to wander blindly in search of the paragraph's topic. In what Dunleavy (2014) calls the "throat clearing" intro, academic writers can begin their paragraphs too broadly as they reference related ideas within the field, making the reader wait until the third or fourth sentence for the main topic. By then, paragraph unity is already threatened, particularly if the reader decided for themselves that something in those first sentences was the topic of interest. To improve a blindfold paragraph, ask yourself if your first few sentences can just be deleted, bringing an existing statement of the main idea into the Topic sentence slot. Remember that the main job of a Topic sentence is "setting the scene" for the reader (Reeves and Leventhal 2012).

17.2.4 The Maze Paragraph

This paragraph has a clear entrance and exit but readers get lost inside it. Sometimes they become so lost that they give up trying to find the logical thread and simply jump to the next paragraph. To improve a maze paragraph, look to the content, number and organization of the Body and Token sentences. Are they all relevant? Is there a logic to their arrangement? Have you signalled the relationships between them with conjunctions (such as 'but', 'or', 'and'), adverbs (such as 'however', 'similarly'), and prepositional phrases (such as 'by contrast', 'in comparison', 'on the other hand')? These little 'connecting' words are essential if your paragraphs are going to "climb the arc", Euchner's (2012) metaphor for strong paragraph development and internal coherence.

17.2.5 The Cliff-Hanger Paragraph

These paragraphs leave the reader in mid-air and jump to the next idea in the argument. Cliff-hangers lack a clear Wrap sentence. In a common example, qualitative research writers often end a paragraph with a quotation. While the right quotation may serve as a Wrap, more often they act as a Token to evidence a specific Body claim. If you want to end with a quotation, ask yourself which function it is serving. Without a Wrap, the writer forfeits two opportunities: both to reinforce what the reader has learned in the paragraph and to signal what is coming next in the argument. Wrap sentences can be used for summary alone or forward signalling; you should consider when each is most effective. Particularly when the next paragraph might otherwise feel like a strange departure from the paper's logical thread, a forward signalling Wrap can smooth this transition.

17.3 Conclusion

Teased out of the writer's subcortex, paragraphing is revealed as not only structure, but also strategy. This chapter offers a model and some general rules for paragraphing, but there is no single right way to paragraph. Models and rules are very helpful to novice writers, but, once learned, they should be treated as a basis for expert improvisation. So don't feel tied down. Try using an abrupt, very short paragraph to highlight a critical moment of transition in your argument. Try dispensing with the declarative Topic sentence in favor of a provocative opening question. Try listing multiple Tokens to give the reader the impression of a wealth of evidence for a particular point. The key to success is to uphold the principles of unity and coherence while you play with strategic paragraphing.

See One, Do One, Teach One
1. Select a paragraph you're struggling with. Apply the concepts of Unity and Coherence to help identify what's going wrong.
2. Use Dunleavy's Topic/Body/Tokens/Wrap model to assess your paragraphs:
   (a) Do you signpost the topic in the first sentence?
   (b) Do your Body sentences develop that topic, or drift off track?
   (c) Have you been strategic about where and why you use Tokens?
   (d) Do you tend to close a paragraph with a Wrap? Does it feel redundant? If so, try a Wrap that includes forward signaling to transition to the next topic.

3. Do you have a recurring paragraphing pitfall? Perhaps you hiccup or create mazes? Identify some pitfall paragraphs and work on improving them. Tip: try listing the claims each paragraph makes in your draft. You may find that some paragraphs make too many points (maze, infinity) while others make

(continued)

very few original points (hiccup). These patterns offer clues about where to direct your attention.

4. Sometimes it can be difficult to see our own paragraphing flaws. Have a colleague read a few pages of your draft with specific attention to the effectiveness of your paragraphs.

References

Dunleavy, P. (2003). *Authoring a PhD*. New York: Palgrave.

Dunleavy, P. (2014, March 26). *How to write paragraphs in research texts*. Medium. https://medium.com/advice-and-help-in-authoring-a-phd-or-non-fiction/how-to-write-paragraphs-80781e2f3054

Euchner, C. (2012). Sentences and paragraphs: Mastering the two most important units of writing. In *The writing minis, book 8*. USA: The New American Press.

Fowler, H. W. (1926). *Modern English usage*. London: Oxford University Press.

Reeves, A., & Leventhal, P. (2012). Paragraphing. *Medical Writing, 21*(4), 298–304. https://doi.org/10.1179/2047480612Z.00000000043.

Chapter 18
Coherence: Keeping the Reader on Track

Readers hunger for coherence.

–Steven Pinker

The effective writer does more than present a succession of well-written sentences or paragraphs. They also control the white space *between* their sentences and paragraphs. Such control transforms a complicated scientific argument into an 'easy read' – not predictable, not without some disruption or surprise, but impossible to get lost in. Writers who achieve this have mastered coherence. This chapter considers how to use the IMRD structure for coherence, how to innovate within that structure without losing the reader, and how to use three metadiscursive moves to keep the reader on track.

Before we get to the white space between your words, however, a quick note about the words themselves. One of the most basic forms of coherence is lexical: using the same words to refer to the same things throughout the story. For instance, if you're writing about "medical error", don't shift your terminology to "clinical failures" or "medical mistakes" in the piece. These are not synonyms, and the subtle changes in meaning will confuse readers. Consistency helps readers stay on track. If you suffer from fear of repetition, don't worry: repetition of key words is the heart of coherence (O'Conner 1999).

18.1 Structure: Convention and Innovation

The first lesson about structure is that you should have one. And, ideally, it should not simply emerge as you write. Go into your writing with a plan. This plan can change if it isn't working, but it shouldn't change by accident. Writing outlines prior to drafting, and revisiting them as the draft matures, is one way to keep yourself thinking about structure.

Most health research manuscripts follow an IMRD structure: they set the stage with an Introduction, explain the Methods of the research, describe the main Results,

L. Lingard, C. Watling, *Story, Not Study: 30 Brief Lessons to Inspire Health Researchers as Writers*, Innovation and Change in Professional Education 19, https://doi.org/10.1007/978-3-030-71363-8_18

and Discuss their implications. Sometimes, though, writers wish to alter the convention. Sword calls such alterations 'hybrid' structures, and many research papers contain at least a few (Sword 2012). Perhaps you wish to include two studies in one paper, requiring paired subsections in Methods and Results. Or maybe your single study asks three, related research questions: you might organize both Methods and Results into three subsections, each addressing one question. Another common example of a hybrid structure relates to the presence and placement of a Theoretical Framework section: do you need one and, if you do, will you position it late in the Introduction or early in the Methods? Limitations sections are also emerging as hybridizations. Traditionally located at the end of the Discussion section, the Limitations can also be found at the beginning of the Discussion or the end of the Methods. Label it, especially if you're placing it somewhere unusual, or readers might miss it. As these examples suggest, "the key to producing a well-structured ...article... is neither slavish imitation nor willful anarchy" (Sword 2012, p. 133). Keep your reader on track by clearly identifying sections and subsections, particularly when you are doing something unexpected.

18.2   Three Metadiscursive Moves

The macro structure of the IMRD's main headings is necessary but not sufficient: readers can still get lost within sections, subsections, and paragraphs. (They can get lost within sentences too; we address that in Chap. 11.) In fact, when you picture your reader, we recommend envisioning an unruly creature – overworked, skimming quickly, difficult to persuade, prone to distraction. In short, apt to wander off the path of your logic at the slightest opportunity. The metadiscursive moves of signposting, pattern and symmetry, and metacommentary can help you keep them in line. By "metadiscursive", we mean words that you use to mark the direction and purpose of the text.

18.2.1   Signposting

Few things are more frustrating to a reader than wondering, "Where is this going?" Regular signposting can prevent this question. Signposting is achieved through headings, subheadings, openers and closers.

The main headings are prescribed for research manuscripts using the IMRD structure, but they don't tell the reader much. You might consider using more descriptive headings. Table 18.1 compares generic and descriptive heading examples:

The descriptive headings offer more detail about the story in each section. You can also try using a colon to combine the generic and the more descriptive: e.g., Introduction: The problem of fatigue. The best headings not only tell the reader what

Table 18.1 Generic and
descriptive headings

Generic headings	Descriptive headings
Introduction	The problem of fatigue
Methods	A phenomenological approach
Results	"Beyond the point of caring"
Discussion	Reconciling fatigue and care

is coming next, they share the writer's thinking process by offering categories, terminology, and conceptual frames (Thomson and Kamler 2013). So choose your headings language carefully.

Even with descriptive headings, however, your sections may be sufficiently long or elaborate that readers will need intermittent guidance to keep on track. Sub-headings address this challenge. Some subheadings are formulaic, such as Methods sections subheadings for "Setting", "Sampling", "Data Collection" and "Data Analysis". You can also create your own. The following subheadings, phrased as questions that are answered in the subsections, lead the reader through the Results of a qualitative study of the care teams for patients with advanced heart failure (HF):

> Who were the patient participants?
> Who did individuals with HF identify as their care team?
> How did individuals with HF conceptualize team members' roles?
> How did team members perceive the patient's role on the team? (LaDonna et al. 2016)

Readers quickly scanning a paper will often use headings and subheadings to get a skeletal sense of the paper's logic. To see if yours are effective, cut and paste them into a blank document: do they represent the main logical steps in the argument? Are they so generic that you can't really tell?

Signposting is also achieved through the explicit use of metadiscursive moves called "openers" and "closers". Linguists call such moves the "discourse about the discourse" (Feak and Swales 2009, p. 38), and they are pervasive in academic writing, most commonly appearing at beginning, ending, and transition points in the argument. Openers are a form of forward signalling, orienting the reader to what's coming in a section or subsection (Thomson and Kamler 2016). Consider this example from the opening paragraph of a Results section:

> Healthcare professionals employed three kinds of humor in their daily work: therapeutic humor, threatening humor and in-my-head humor. In what follows, we will briefly describe each type, illustrate it with examples from the fieldnotes, and use interview data to suggest what motivates its use.

This opener tells the reader how many subsections are coming (three), explains which data will appear as evidence (fieldnotes and interview transcripts), and fore-shadows that motivation will be addressed as a core idea. Opener language uses phrases such as "In what follows", "This section describes", "Below we present", or more elaborate signposts such as "We will explore…beginning with…and then considering…".

Closers, or backward signalling, are moves that occur at the end of a section or subsection and tell the reader what to take away from what they have read (Thomson and Kamler 2016). They may also anticipate what is coming next. The same Results section might end with:

> As these results suggest, humor is multifaceted, tied to context, and dependent on relation-ships for its meaning and impact. Even 'in-my-head' humor is not detached from these influences, which has implications for how educators might harness (or hinder) the social-izing power of humor in clinical situations.

As a closer, these sentences summarize the main points and foreshadow the focus of the Discussion: the question of what these results mean for addressing humor as a socializing force.

Openers and closers are important not only at the section and subsection levels; as Chap. 17 explained, paragraphs also include these features. Topic sentences serve as openers, signalling the main idea that the paragraph will explore, and Wrap sentences summarize the current paragraph and anticipate its connection to the next.

You can go too far with Signposting, boring or confusing your reader. You will bore them if you "unthinkingly follow the advice to say what you're going to say, say it, and then say what you've said" (Pinker 2014, p. 38). This advice is more appropriate to oratory than it is to prose. You will confuse them if your signposts are burdensome or illogical, "like complicated directions for a shortcut which take longer to figure out than the time the short cut would save" (Pinker 2014, p. 39). Confusion can also arise from too many headings, which can break up the forward motion of the argument by reducing the transition work at the sentence and para-graph level. By expecting the headings to do the work for you, your transitions remain implicit. Ensure that your openers and closers are guiding around the headings, and limit the subheading levels to what is essential.

18.2.2 Pattern and Symmetry

Another metadiscursive move takes advantage of reader's expectations by using patterns and symmetry to organize material. Logical patterns – general to specific, big to small, old to new, pro to con, least to most important/valuable/controversial, etc. – set up a recognizable map that guides readers. Patterns only work, however, when you follow them precisely. A disrupted pattern confuses the reader, as does a forgotten one. Therefore, when you are reviewing your prose, check that the pattern remains consistent. And if it stretches over a long section of prose, explicitly re-invoke it at regular intervals using phrases such as: "A more controversial issue is", "More recently", "Even more specifically", etc. Finally, if you are overlaying multiple patterns, do so explicitly and carefully:

> The definition of medical error has shifted significantly from the late 1990s to present day. Temporal changes are not the only ones worth noting, however; definitions can also be mapped on a spectrum of positivist to constructivist ontology. And the ontological shifts correspond with temporal ones in surprising ways.

In this example, the first sentence functions as a closer, summarizing the temporal pattern used up to this point in the literature review. The next sentence introduces the next pattern – from positivist to constructivist ontology – and foreshadows that the relationship between the two patterns will also be considered.

Symmetry also draws on the reader's expectations to create coherence. Symmetry is achieved by repeating structures throughout the manuscript. For instance, the earlier example of using questions as subheadings in the Results section achieves symmetry: if one of the subheadings were *not* a question, symmetry would be lost. Symmetry can also cut across manuscript sections: one of our favourite grant-writing techniques, for instance, is to establish an order for the study objectives (e.g., 1, 2, 3) and maintain that order throughout all sections. In this approach, Methods is organized according to those procedures related to Objectives 1, 2, and 3, and Anticipated Challenges and Expected Outcomes are also organized in terms of those relating to Objectives 1, 2, and 3. This can be an effective way of keeping a reader on track when a study is multi-faceted.

18.2.3   Metacommentary

Research writing is full of metacommentary. As Graff and Birkenstein (2014) put it, you're actually writing "two texts joined at the hip: one makes the argument, the other ensures your argument isn't mistaken for one you don't want to make" (p. 130). This is an essential strategy to master "because the written word is prone to so much mischief and can be interpreted in so many different ways, we need metacommentary to keep misinterpretations and other communication misfires at bay" (p. 131).

Writers use metacommentary to clarify, elaborate, affiliate, justify, acknowledge, deflect, anticipate and answer objections. Table 18.2 offers examples, with explicit *translations* of what the metacommentary implies:

As the translations suggest, coherence is strengthened when you imagine yourself in conversation with a reader. Not all readers are created equal, however, so it can be helpful to imagine a complete set of what we call "barometer" readers: a revered icon of the field, a wide-eyed novice, a representative of an enemy camp, a curious layperson, an expert from an adjacent field who is passing through. The type and degree of metacommentary will vary for each of these readers, such that what is necessary guidance for one may seem like manipulation to another (Hyland 2017). Decide who your main audience is and aim for coherence in their reading experience. You can nod to other readers periodically, for instance by providing definitions for terms a novice or layperson might misunderstand, but keep your primary conversant in the foreground.

Table 18.2 Metacommentary with translations

Purpose	Example	Translation
To clarify	In using the term "failure" rather than "error", we intend…	*Dear Reader, let us explain our terminology*
To elaborate, to justify	This sampling method offered a number of advantages that offset its drawbacks…	*Dear Reader, you may be worried about the limits of this sampling approach. Let us elaborate*
To affiliate	Drawing on the work of educators who have created a model of "productive failure", we …	*Dear Reader, our approach is based on other scholars who have come before and whom you may recognize as credible*
To acknowledge	While other fields have made recent advances in the science of big data, medical education…	*Dear Reader, in case you were wondering whether we are aware of scholarship in other fields, we reference it here*
To anticipate	Critical feminist scholars might take a different view of this problem	*Dear Reader, we recognize that there is more than one way to approach this issue*
To anticipate & answer objections	Although it has been argued that interview data is irretrievably subjective, we contend …	*Dear Reader, we are aware that there is controversy in the field, and we align ourselves consciously*

18.3   Conclusion

As Pinker (2014) has noted, "so eager are readers to seek coherence that they will often supply it when none exists" (p. 141). Don't leave the story to the unruly reader – who knows what they might come up with in the white space between your sentences, paragraphs, and sections? Control that white space and create coherence in your manuscript by planning for structure and mastering the main metadiscursive moves.

See One, Do One, Teach One
1. Cut and paste the headings and subheadings from your draft into a new Word document. Do they express all the key steps in your logic?
2. Review your paper for openers and closers:

   (a) Do they appear at major transitions to help the reader?
   (b) Do they feel sufficient? Do any seem redundant?

3. Have you used pattern or symmetry in your paper? If so, are you consistent? Is it the best pattern for your argument?
4. Create a set of barometer readers for your current manuscript. Name them so that you can picture a conversation with them.

(continued)

5. Identify places where you have used metacommentary:

   (a) Translate it: what are you telling the reader?
   (b) Consider how you might tailor the type and amount of metacommentary for each barometer reader.

References

Feak, C. B., & Swales, J. M. (2009). *Telling a research story: Writing a literature review*. Ann Arbor: University of Michigan Press.

Graff, G., & Birkenstein, C. (2014). *They say, I say: The moves that matter in academic writing*. New York: W.W. Norton.

Hyland, K. (2017). Metadiscourse: What is it and where is it going? *Journal of Pragmatics, 113*, 16–29. https://doi.org/10.1016/j.pragma.2017.03.007.

LaDonna, K. A., Bates, J., Tait, G. R., McDougall, A., Schulz, V., & Lingard, L. (2016). 'Who is on your health-care team?' Asking individuals with heart failure about care team membership and roles. *Health Expectations, 20*(2), 198–210. https://doi.org/10.1111/hex.12447.

O'Conner, P. T. (1999). *Words fail me: What everyone who writes should know about writing*. New York: Harcourt.

Pinker, S. (2014). *The sense of style: The thinking person's guide to writing in the 21st century*. New York: Viking.

Sword, H. (2012). *Stylish academic writing*. Cambridge, MA: Harvard University Press.

Thomson, P., & Kamler, B. (2013). *Writing for peer-reviewed journals: Strategies for getting published*. London: Routledge.

Thomson, P., & Kamler, B. (2016). *Detox your writing: Strategies for doctoral researchers*. London: Routledge.

Chapter 19
The Three "S"s of Editing: Story, Structure, and Style

Editing can be a fight. Wrestling a meandering draft into a concise, publishable paper challenges even seasoned writers. Editing means shaping and fine-tuning the raw materials of that imperfect draft into a strong final product. Done well, editing focuses and elevates your writing. Done poorly, editing risks endless loops of revisions that can leave you wondering whether you are strengthening the work at all.

You need a plan – a systematic approach to editing. To ensure that your editing boosts the quality of your work, remember to attend to the three "S"s: story, structure, and style. Of course, story deserves some attention before you write a single word, and structure and style considerations will naturally arise as you write your draft. Too much in-the-moment editing, however, can stifle your writing momentum. Draft something first, then use this approach to ensure you've said what you really want to say.

19.1 Edit at the Level of the Paper: Think *Story*

Your paper must tell a persuasive and compelling story. When editing for story, think about your target journal and its likely readers. Who are they, what do they care about, and what do they already know about the problem your study addresses? Typically, medical journals favor concise, pragmatic stories; their readers want to know how they can use research findings, or how those findings will shape their practice. But readers of a theoretically-oriented education journal might want to know how your work challenges or elaborates existing understandings of a concept or problem. Different stories work for different audiences.

Originality looms large in publication decisions. Papers that are clearly written and methodologically rigorous may well be rejected if they fail to persuade reviewers and editors that they have something new to say. Your story, therefore,

© The Author(s), under exclusive license to Springer Nature Switzerland AG 2021   127
L. Lingard, C. Watling, *Story, Not Study: 30 Brief Lessons to Inspire Health Researchers as Writers*, Innovation and Change in Professional Education 19,
https://doi.org/10.1007/978-3-030-71363-8_19

needs to highlight how the work builds, advances, or deepens knowledge in the field. Don't over-reach, but don't suffer false modesty either. Remember that the articulation of your story's hook in the paper's introduction must be more than empty rhetoric. It is a promise that the work will matter, and in the Discussion you'll need to deliver on that promise.

Avoid the traps that derail good research stories. Although researchers embark on an intellectual journey in completing a study, readers need not be dragged through all the twists and turns of that journey. Tell your story coherently, not necessarily chronologically. Limit jargon. Unless you intend to write solely for your field's insiders, be kind to your readers and explain terms that may be unfamiliar. Once you have defined your terms, ensure that you use them consistently throughout your paper. Hearkening back to the drama metaphor we used in Chap. 7, don't give your characters new names halfway through the story. Beware of throwaway references to theory; ground your story in theory when it makes narrative sense to do so. And resist becoming too attached – to a paragraph, a sentence, a result, even a turn of phrase. Sometimes the best edits begin with the courage to try a revision that deletes something you like, but that you feel in your gut doesn't belong.

19.2 Edit at the Level of the Paragraph: Think *Structure*

Chapter 17 offers reminders on strong paragraph construction, and it may be useful to review these when editing your paper for structure. Remember that good research stories thrive on a logical flow of ideas. Paragraphs are the structural foundation of any paper, and their arrangement and composition dictate how readily readers will be able to follow your logic. Each paragraph should be a coherent unit, addressing one topic. Beware of both long paragraphs that tilt from one idea to another, and also of single-sentence paragraphs that fail to adequately develop an idea.

Start each paragraph with a topic sentence that flags what is to come for readers, and then ensure that the paragraph is true to the spirit of that sentence. Think about transitions between paragraphs, and compose topic sentences to show readers how what has gone before relates to what will come next. Consider this transitional topic sentence:

> This exploration of how students interpret and use feedback is illuminating, but its focus on the individual learner without reference to the learning environment is limiting.

This sentence signals a shift in topic, from the cognitive (how individuals make sense of feedback) to the sociocultural (how the learning environment shapes the feedback process). It prepares readers that they are about to be presented with a new wrinkle that they perhaps hadn't considered, explicitly signposting the change in focus. Transitions need not always be elaborate; sometimes a word ("Conversely...") or phrase ("But this research overlooks a critical issue...") is sufficient.

A struggle to link paragraphs convincingly can be a symptom of faulty composition. Consider, when transitions prove challenging, whether paragraphs are in the wrong place, or whether one paragraph doesn't belong. A place that is difficult to get readers to and from perhaps doesn't need to be visited at all.

19.3 Edit at the Level of the Sentence: Think *Style*

Sentence-level editing should make the incorrect correct – fixing grammatical errors – but it should also aim to make the correct better by attending to style. Effective sentence-level editing requires us to recognize when sentences are awkward or unclear, to identify the source of that awkwardness, and to deploy a range of remedies. Entire books promise to build these critical skills so that writers can inject polish and style into their writing. Here, we offer only three key pieces of advice: power up your verbs, prune needless words and limit nominalizations.

19.3.1 Power Up Your Verbs

Verbs are the engines of our stories; they're so important that we've dedicated a whole chapter to them (Chap. 12). Successful editing puts those lessons into action. Look for opportunities to replace weak verbs with more robust, action-oriented ones. Consider this sentence:

> When feedback negatively **affects** self-esteem or **makes** the recipient emotional, its potential usefulness may be lost.

While grammatically correct, the sentence features two milquetoast verbs (affects and makes) that diminish its power. Here's a stronger version of the same sentence, enhanced by swapping out weak verbs for stronger ones:

> When feedback **threatens** self-esteem or **stirs** strong emotions, its potential usefulness may be lost.

Forms of the verb "to be" (is, are, was, were, be been) often underperform in sentences, and cry out for strengthening. For example:

> Stress **is** a frequent problem facing medical students.

might be re-crafted for greater impact:

> Stress **plagues** medical students.

Be bold in your verb choices. Though you may sometimes be chastened by reviewers if you've stepped over the line, you might be surprised at the positive impact of just the right verb. Here's one of our favorite examples:

> Lack of continuity **bedevils** the undergraduate clinical teaching environment to the detriment of student learning (Bates et al. 2013).

The dramatic (but spot-on) verb choice grabs the reader's attention in a way that saying "lack of continuity is a problem" just wouldn't have done. Of course, one can probably only use the verb "bedevil" once in a career!

19.3.2   Prune Needless Words

Identify and eliminate unnecessary words and redundant phrases. Ask: can I get my point across with fewer words? Almost always, less will be more. Pinker (2014) has compiled helpful lists of what he calls "morbidly obese phrases" (p.104); writers would do well to affix these to their computer screens while they edit. Some of these phrases can be replaced with leaner equivalents; for example, substituting "if" for "in the event that" or "we must" for "it is imperative that we" (p. 105). Other bloated phrases can simply be eliminated altogether; "it is a well-known fact that" need never start a sentence, for example. Unless your purpose is to suggest that no one could possibly hold a dissenting opinion – think Jane Austen's famous opener, "It is a truth universally acknowledged, that a single man in possession of a good fortune must be in want of a wife" (as cited in Fish 2011).

Constructions involving "it", "this", "that", and "there" invite our editorial attention also. These constructions contribute to what Helen Sword calls "flabby prose" (Sword, n.d.). Consider:

There are many faculty members who are frustrated by the limited time that they have available for teaching.

This flabby sentence can be pared down significantly:

Lack of time frustrates many faculty teachers.

Pared-down prose is not just shorter; it is more powerful. Consider these sequential edits:

A well-known business fact is that alignment with partners and communities must be rooted in high brand awareness.

Alignment with partners and communities must be rooted in high brand awareness.

In business, brand awareness is foundational.

The first edit targets what Lanham (2007, p. 13) calls the "'Blah blah is that' opening" and removes "A well-known business fact is. . .". The second edit is more substantive, and requires asking the question "What am I trying to say anyway?" That prompt is useful when simply removing a few words doesn't seem to do the job.

Finally, train your editorial attention to adverbs. We can often render these verb modifiers obsolete by choosing stronger, more evocative verbs (see also Chap. 16). Compare these examples:

Educators **strongly recommend** feedback as an essential and indispensable element of clinical learning.

Educators **champion** feedback's indispensable role in clinical learning.

Note that we have not only substituted the verb "champion" for the weaker phrase "strongly recommend", but we have also eliminated the word "essential", which is rendered redundant by the stronger "indispensable."

19.3.3   Limit Nominalizations

Nominalizations are nouns formed from other parts of speech, especially verbs. Academic writing overflows with words like "contribution", "participation", "development", and "indication". Buried in these familiar nouns are active verbs – "contribute", "participate", "develop", "indicate" – whose power has been neutralized by reconstituting them as nouns. Sword (2012) calls nominalizations "zombie nouns", and explains that their impact is to weigh down prose, sapping its energy and verve. When editing, root out these deadweights whenever possible. Consider the difference between the following two sentences:

The learning process involves the initial **demonstration** of skills in a simulated setting, followed by the **application** of those skills to a real clinical situation.

Learners must first **demonstrate** skills in a simulated setting, then **apply** those skills to a real clinical situation.

A nominalization typically contains the verb you need to enliven your sentence; the editing trick is to liberate it.

19.3.4   Conclusion

Editing requires writers to critically assess their own work as a prelude to improving it – no easy feat. We suggest three productive strategies to address this challenge: (1) read your work aloud, which helps you to think like a reader rather than a writer, (2) allow a gap between writing the draft and editing it, which softens your attachment to words and phrases that might need to be discarded, and (3) invite a few colleagues and friends to weigh in, supplementing your self-assessment with voices of reason. But while critical self-assessment is productive, perfectionism is not. Editing can continue indefinitely; much published work could have been improved further. At some point – for your own sanity and for submission – you must be able to say "good enough".

At least until you receive the reviews.

See One, Do One, Teach One

1. Identify opportunities for productive edits in a paragraph you're working on. Highlight each of the following:

   (a) Forms of the verb 'to be'
   (b) Redundant phrases
   (c) Modifiers (adjectives and adverbs)
   (d) Nominalizations

2. Now try to exploit some of these opportunities. Can you replace a "to be" verb with something stronger? Can you snip out some needless words? How many of the modifiers are unnecessary? Which nominalizations are improved by liberating the verbs they contain?

3. When you're asked to give feedback to a student or colleague on their writing, try to be specific in how you label the issues you identify:

   (a) At the level of story, does the originality of the work shine through?
   (b) At the level of structure, do the paragraphs link together logically?
   (c) At the level of style, can you name the problems explicitly and suggest some fixes?

References

Bates, J., Konkin, K., Suddards, C., Dobson, S., & Pratt, D. (2013). Student perceptions of assessment and feedback in longitudinal integrated clerkships. *Medical Education, 47*(4), 362–374. https://doi.org/10.1111/medu.12087.

Fish, S. (2011). *How to write a sentence and how to read one*. New York: Harper.

Lanham, R. A. (2007). *Revising prose*. New York: Pearson Longman.

Pinker, S. (2014). *The sense of style*. New York: Viking.

Sword, H. (2012, July 23). Zombie nouns. *The New York Times*. https://opinionator.blogs.nytimes.com/2012/07/23/zombie-nouns/. Accessed 8 Sept 2020.

Sword, H. (n.d.). *The writer's diet*. http://writersdiet.com/. Accessed 24 Sept 2020.

Chapter 20
Pace, Pause, & Silence: Creating Emphasis & Suspense in Your Writing

Well-timed silence *hath more eloquence than* speech.

–Martin Tupper

Winston Churchill is said to have annotated his speeches with reminders to himself about rhythm and tempo – when to be silent, when to appear to struggle for the right word, when to pause for audience response (whether heckling or applause). His oratory, as a consequence, felt more like psalm than prose. Like other effective public speakers, Churchill knew that what is *not* said impacts the audience as much as what is. A pregnant pause whets appetites. An unanswered question hangs heavily. An abrupt redirection defers logical resolution. Wouldn't it be lovely if writing could offer the same possibility?

It can. Prose need not always be a fast-flowing faucet, and readers need not be continuously engulfed. When we use pace, pause and silence strategically, we can craft a text that engages readers. This chapter describes how to use punctuation and sentence structure to create emphasis and suspense in your research writing.

20.1 Punctuation

Punctuation is not only grammatical; it is also rhetorical. You can use it for persuasion, to shape the reader's experience. Because all forms of punctuation temper the forward motion of your prose, they are tools for pacing and silence, for producing anticipation and resolution, curiosity and satisfaction. Periods and exclamation points are the strongest punctuation, bringing the reader to a complete stop, a sense of an idea resolved. While a question mark creates a complete stop, it has the opposite effect. It implies an answer, creating a moment of silence in the prose that produces suspense. You can extend that silence, perhaps by ending the paragraph with a question and answering it in the next paragraph. Or you can shorten the silence by providing an immediate answer:

L. Lingard, C. Watling, *Story, Not Study: 30 Brief Lessons to Inspire Health Researchers as Writers*, Innovation and Change in Professional Education 19, https://doi.org/10.1007/978-3-030-71363-8_20

Too often, our development as writers relies on trial and error, haphazard feedback, accidental improvements. Sad, but does it matter?

Too often, our development as writers relies on trial and error, haphazard feedback, accidental improvements. Sad, but does it matter? Only if we hope to find joy in our work.

Such use of questions can feel conversational, which is an effective strategy for engaging the reader. But it may take manuscript reviewers aback. Therefore, use them sparingly, probably not more than once in a piece of writing. Recently, a writing team we're part of realized the line had been crossed when we received the following reviewer comment: "Avoid asking a series of questions without answering these, see p. 4, lines 14–15."

Colons also allow you to instill anticipation: they're like an intake of breath before revealing an illustration or a list. The ellipsis creates a drifting pause but … likely an unusual technique to find in a scholarly manuscript. Commas and semi-colons are a lighter harness but still curb the headlong flow of your prose (Truss 2003). Commas, with their origins in antiquity and the elocutional school of punctuation, indicate intonation and pauses in oral speech, and they retain some of this flavor in writing (Crystal 2015). (See also Chap. 14.) Semi-colons in particular help signal shifts in logic. Used properly, they tell the reader to gather herself for a development; however, used poorly, they send her on fruitless searches for mid-sentence meaning. Consider this sentence:

Work-based learning is central to postgraduate medical education; ethical issues rarely get attention.

Here, the semi-colon presents a moment of intense work for the reader, who must ascertain what ethical issues have to do with the centrality of work-based learning in postgraduate medical education. The semi-colon's promise of logical development remains unfulfilled and the reader is left wondering. *That* kind of pause you don't want to cultivate.

Punctuating for pace is also a way to establish a particular writer's voice in a piece. Seeking drama? Try short sentences. Their strong, staccato pacing results as much from the pauses between them as from their brevity. Trying for a conversational tone? Brackets take the reader on a brief detour from the main idea and create a sense of (hopefully purposeful) meandering. Similarly, the em dash – famously loved or hated – takes a momentary sidestep away from the main logic. Use it to set up whispered asides or provocative barbs. Take care though: brackets and dashes are boutique punctuation tools that can annoy the reader. Brackets, because they leave the reader to infer how the bracketed material integrates into the argument, can imply lazy thinking if you overuse them. Ask a trusted reader for honest feedback if you have tried to use punctuation for rhetorical effect and you wonder if you might have crossed the line. Visit Chap. 23 for more on establishing your writer's voice.

20.2 Syntax

Syntax is the set of rules, principles, and processes that govern how we construct sentences. Three aspects of syntax – sentence structure, subject-verb placement, and word order inversion – are described below as tools for pacing and emphasis.

First, you can employ sentence types to control the pacing of your prose. In Chap. 11, we considered the structure and purposes of three sentence types: simple, compound and complex. Consider this example:

> My scholarly life is inextricably bound up with words. I write them to understand my research results. I read them to cultivate my ideas. I speak them to engage my colleagues. I publish them to share my knowledge.

Because all of these sentences are simple in their structure, there is a sense of strong, regular pacing. Parallel structure enhances this pacing by creating a metronomic rhythm through the repeating subject-verb-object construction: "I write them," "I read them", "I speak them", "I publish them". Of course, you can't continue ad nauseam in this pacing or your prose will sound like a primary school, Dick-and-Jane reader, plodding along rather than marching ahead. Pacing only works rhetorically when it is purposeful and varied. So perhaps we should quicken the pace in the next sentence by distilling the parallel structure down to two parallel lists of verbs:

> My scholarly life is inextricably bound up with words. I write them to understand my research results. I read them to cultivate my ideas. I speak them to engage my colleagues. I publish them to share my knowledge. I love, covet and despise them; I create, destroy and mourn them.

It is not so much the simple sentence structure in this example that creates the pacing, it is the combination of simple structure, parallelism and distilling of the pattern.

Sentence structure doesn't *dictate* pace; it's a tool you use to *create* pace. Consider the following three sentences. They are all complex in structure, which means they have a main clause and a subordinate clause. The subordinate clause is just that – it is subordinate to, its information assigned less importance than that in the main clause. The subordinate clause is also transportable: you can put it at the beginning, the end, or somewhere mid-sentence.

> Systematic reviews remain the gold standard review methodology in health research, although we increasingly recognize their limitations.

> Although we increasingly recognize their limitations, systematic reviews remain the gold standard review methodology in health research.

> Systematic reviews, although we increasingly recognize their limitations, remain the gold standard review methodology in health research.

The decision about how to position the two clauses should not be random. Rather, it should reflect the "given-new principle" governing the ordering of information in a sentence, which states that known (given) information should precede new in order to maximize cohesion (Halliday and Matthiessen 2004). Each of the above examples, therefore, suggests a different assumption about what the reader already knows, and what is new to them. If we make such assumptions consciously as writers, we can play with emphasis and suspense.

Another method to create emphasis in your writing is by altering conventional subject/verb positioning. In English, the **subject** and the **verb** are the dominant meaning slots in the sentence, and the convention is to place them side by side in order to decrease the reader's cognitive load. This example follows that convention:

> **Qualitative research methods** have become a popular approach to knowledge creation in our field.

Every convention, however, presents a rhetorical opportunity to improvise for effect. Williams (1990) calls these "artful interruptions" (p. 159). Purposefully separating the subject and verb can create emphasis because the inserted phrase elaborates on the just-introduced subject, insisting the reader pause there rather than immediately landing on the verb. Consider this example:

> **Qualitative research methods**, rare twenty years ago in health services research, **have become** a popular approach to knowledge creation in our field.

Be careful not to create too much distance between subject and verb when you use this technique. As Sword (2012) cautions, more than a dozen words between subject and verb can confuse readers.

Another way to play with syntax for emphasis is word order inversion. Every language falls into one of six word-order types (Dryer 2012). English belongs to the *subject*-**verb**-*object* type, in which the natural order is to place the subject first, as this example illustrates:

> **We value** *reliability and validity* above all else in high stakes assessments.

If you alter that order, referred to as 'inversion', you change the emphasis in the sentence:

> *Reliability and validity* **we value** above all else in high stakes assessments.

When you invert subject-verb-object word order, listen carefully for what happens to tone:

> We need to change if our educational practices are going to embrace medicine's humanity. And **change** *we* **will**.

This example moves part of the verb before the subject to emphasize the word "change". But it perhaps sounds a bit … archaic? Yoda-esque? Knowing some of the more common uses of inversion can help you adopt this technique without just sounding odd. Inversion is used with negative adverbs:

> Rarely **does** *the health professions education literature* position itself socio-historically.

It may also be used when a sentence starts with an adverbial expression of place:

From the sciences **comes** *our expectation of objectivity*; from the humanities **comes** *our embrace of subjectivity*.

Inversion is how we create questions:

Are *entrustment decisions* more reliable than conventional assessments?

And it is used with "so + adjective" constructions:

So ubiquitous **is** *the call for more direct observation*, that the act of questioning its feasibility in clinical training seems somewhat sacrilegious.

Because each of these inversion techniques works implicitly, through the *absence* of an expected pattern, they offer tools for creating subtle emphasis.

20.3 Conclusion

Pace, pause and silence are important tools in your writing. Knowing the conventions of punctuation and syntax allows you to bend them strategically. Such bending can both help your readers pay attention and enlist them into productive engagement with your ideas. Remember though, there is a fine line between cultivating a curious, engaged reader and creating a frustrated, disengaged one. These are delicate aspects of the writer's craft. Use them wisely.

See One, Do One, Teach One
1. Scan your draft and take an inventory of your punctuation.
   (a) What forms do you repeatedly use? Commas and periods should be common; em dashes, question and exclamation marks should not.
   (b) What punctuation have you not used at all? Why not? Give it a try. For instance, consider whether there is one place in your manuscript where a question mark could be effective.
2. Looking at one page of your manuscript, assess your use of simple, compound and complex sentences. Revise for variety if you find you tend to write mostly simple or mostly complex sentences.
3. Select some complex sentences for analysis. Where is the subordinate clause? Does its placement reflect the given/new principle, and, if not, have you flaunted that principle purposefully and to good effect?

References

Crystal, D. (2015). *Making a point: The persnickety story of English punctuation.* New York: St. Martin's Press.

Dryer, M. S. (2012). Order of subject, object and verb. In M. S. Dryer & M. Haspelmath (Eds.), *The world atlas of language structures online.* Max Planck Institute for Evolutionary Anthropology. http://wals.info/chapter/81. Accessed 11 Sept 2020.

Halliday, M. A. K., & Matthiessen, C. (2004). *An introduction to functional grammar* (3rd ed.). London: Arnold.

Sword, H. (2012). *Stylish academic writing.* Cambridge, MA: Harvard University Press.

Truss, L. (2003). *Eats, shoots & leaves: The zero tolerance approach to punctuation.* London: Profile Books.

Williams, J. M. (1990). *Style: Toward clarity and grace.* Chicago: University of Chicago Press.

Chapter 21
The Academic Hedge, Part I:
Modal Tuning in Your Research Writing

The cautious seldom err.

–Confucius

One of the reasons academic conferences are so popular (in addition to geography and climate) is that interacting with other researchers 'in the flesh' can be great fun. Especially outside the formal program, in the cafés and bars of the conference city. Over tiny Dutch coffees or goblets of Spanish wine, scholars share the latest twists and turns, successes and sufferings, agreements and arguments in the field. They laugh, they contradict, they argue – mostly with collegial vigor! But have you ever wondered, opening the latest issue of a journal, what's happened to these dynamic, engaging conversationalists? Why do they seem to be "writing without conviction" (Hyland 1996)?

Researchers can seem quite mincing and modest creatures in their writing. They follow an implicit set of linguistic conventions to represent themselves as cautious, even uncertain as they critique existing knowledge and offer their own knowledge claims. This is the "academic hedge", regarded as critical to scientific discourse and readily (even unconsciously) performed by the experienced writer, but difficult to reproduce for the novice or the non-native English writer (Chen 2010; Yang et al. 2015). When should your writing express confidence, and when should it be tentative? When should you be assertive, and when deferential? Too little hedging, and you can come across as naïve, brash, even rude. Too much, and you can sound as if you don't have control of the literature, or you don't believe your own results. The next two chapters introduce epistemic modality and politeness theory in order to help you to use the academic hedge skillfully.

L. Lingard, C. Watling, *Story, Not Study: 30 Brief Lessons to Inspire Health Researchers as Writers*, Innovation and Change in Professional Education 19, https://doi.org/10.1007/978-3-030-71363-8_21

21.1   Tools for Expressing Epistemic Modality

Writers express their judgement about the degree of probability or factual status of a proposition by using "epistemic modality". In research writing, where ideas – particularly new ones – are only ordained as knowledge by community consensus, a robust set of tools exists to express degrees of probability and factual status. The six sentences in Table 21.1 illustrate this spectrum, from weakest to strongest probability:

Epistemic modality is produced through modal auxiliary (helper) verbs (e.g., may, might, must) and adverbs (e.g., possibly, probably, certainly), as well as through lexical (main) verbs that express degrees of certainty (e.g., wonder, think, believe, know). Expressions that weaken probability are also referred to as 'hedges', and those that strengthen probability are referred to as "boosters" (Hyland 1998).

We could add two more columns to this table. On the far left side, an even more speculative or hedged expression would be a question: "Is it true that social media has influenced anti-vaccination rates?" On the far right side, the strongest expression would not be marked by modality at all: "Social media has influenced anti-vaccination rates." When there is no modality present, as in this last example, the writer is making no claim to knowledge; instead, this sentence represents the invocation of common knowledge (Myers 1989). Even a booster weakens the claim: "Certainly social media has influenced anti-vaccination rates" is actually a less strong claim than if the booster "certainly" were removed.

Table 21.2 offers a partial list of modal verbs and adverbs that you can use to express degrees of possibility and certainty in your writing:

A key function of epistemic modality is to indicate the degree of certainty of a proposition and the writer's confidence in it. It offers, therefore, an essential tool when you are reviewing the literature and mapping the gap that your own work will fill. Modality is not a simple recipe, however. It is relational and contextual; therefore, many of the words in Table 21.2 can shift category, as the examples that follow in this chapter will illustrate.

Table 21.1   Epistemic modality spectrum

It may be true that social media has influenced anti-vaccination rates	I wonder if it is true that social media has influenced anti-vaccination rates	It is probably true that social media has influenced anti-vaccination rates	I think it is true that social media has influenced anti-vaccination rates	It must be true that social media has influenced anti-vaccination rates	It is certainly true social media has influenced anti-vaccination rates
Weak/speculative		Intermediary/probabilitive		Strong/assertive	

Table 21.2 Selected verbs and adverbs to express epistemic modality

Certainty	Auxiliary verbs	Lexical verbs	Modal adverbs
Strong	Will, cannot, must	Know, understand, argue, affirm, stress, emphasize, maintain, declare, stipulate, explain, warn, conclude, clarify, identify, insist	Undoubtedly, always, never, definitely, clearly, certainly, obviously, entirely, completely, increasingly
Moderate	Should, would, can, ought to, tends to	Comment, explain, indicate, note, observe, state, describe, identify, find, show, suggest	Usually, likely, probably, regularly, generally, often, frequently, rarely, typically, over the past decade
Weak	May, might, could	Speculate, wonder, believe, note, offer, view, suspect, suggest, consider, propose, debate	Possibly, conceivably, occasionally, tentatively, perhaps, maybe, recently, less, currently, apparently, reportedly

21.2 Tuning Modality Up and Down

The good news about this is that it allows writers to project nuanced degrees of certainty. The bad news is that, if you're not careful, you can express strong or weak certainty when you don't intend it. Restricting yourself to verbs and adverbs in the "moderate" category isn't a solution. This can create limp writing, in which you appear to be simply summarizing knowledge rather than evaluating and controlling it to create an argument. Instead, think carefully about how you are putting together a variety of modal words in your sentences.

Combinations are the key to nuanced author positioning. For instance, you can combine a verb expressing strong certainty with an adverb that weakens it: "Researchers have tentatively concluded that". Or you can strengthen a moderate verb with an adverb projecting more certainty: "Health policy researchers increasingly find". Adverbs of time also have shifting meanings: "Recently, a review suggested that" can project stronger certainty because the knowledge is very current, or weaker certainty because the knowledge has yet to gain the community's approval, signalled by others taking up the knowledge and reproducing it over time.

Given this complexity, how should the careful writer proceed? Overall, think of 'tuning' your certainty up and down, like the volume knob on an old stereo. First, ask yourself whether you have strong, moderate or weak certainty in a knowledge claim you are reviewing or making, and then tune it accordingly. For instance, you can use verbs that signal strong certainty when you are summarizing well-accepted knowledge in your field:

Clinical teaching **requires** a balance of patient safety and learner development.

Expressed with such certainty, this claim appears to be common knowledge; it may not even need a reference. If that seems too certain, then locating or attributing that knowledge is a way to tune the certainty down just a bit. The example below achieves this by locating the knowledge in time and attributing it to a group:

Over the past decade, researchers have described clinical teaching as requiring a balance of patient safety and learner development.

You can further tune the certainty up or down by altering the temporal reference. "*Recently*, researchers have described. . ." would weaken the expression of certainty, while "*A generation of* research has described. . ." would strengthen it. Here is another example that alters the certainty of the initial claim:

Sociological research demonstrates that clinical teaching requires a balance of patient safety and learner development.

In this second example, "Sociological research" is an attribution to a scholarly field that lessens the certainty. Attributions lessen certainty because they retain the flavour of a knowledge *claim*; as Myers (1989) points out, any reference to a source lessens the factual status of a claim, even when that source is well-regarded. However, in this instance, the claim retains its sense of certainty because of the verb "demonstrates". Choosing another verb, such as "suggests" or "proposes", would tune the certainty down even further, as would citing a person rather than a whole discipline, as in "*Carruthers et al* demonstrate".

21.3   Expressing Uncertainty

The whole point of doing, and publishing, research is to work in the spaces of moderate and weak certainty: things we do not yet know for sure, expressions of new ideas, debates about alternative conceptualizations. This is why you need to become fluent in weaving together different degrees of modality and, in particular, carefully expressing moderate and weak modality: not because others' ideas are wrong, but because we are all engaged in a conversation to continuously refine and advance a body of knowledge. Consider how the following passage marks summaries of existing knowledge with modality. We have highlighted verb and adverb constructions that project **strong**, moderate and *weak* degrees of certainty as the writers state the problem and gap that their work addresses:

To be a student in medical school *may be* stressful[1-3]. Previous studies have shown relatively high levels of distress, such as symptoms of depression[4,5] and suicidal thoughts [6,7] in medical undergraduates. Less is known about what conditions encourage positive mental health, and a recent review of research on medical student distress **emphasised** the need for research concerning the factors that promote well-being[8]. Despite increased attention being paid to positive psychological health and well-being **during the past decades**[9,10], *only a few* studies have focused on life satisfaction and coping in medical students. Of these, one study found that problem focused and emotion focused coping related positively to physical health in first year medical students[11], and another study found that coping strategies characterised by engagement predicted fewer symptoms of depression compared to disengagement strategies[12]. A qualitative study of medical student perceptions of an elective wellness course reported positive responses from the students[13]. A *recent* study **concluded** that personal statements and referees' reports used in medical school applications **cannot** predict who will be satisfied or dissatisfied with a medical career[14]. To date, **no** longitudinal study has identified predictors of sustained high levels of life satisfaction among medical students (Kjeldstadli et al. 2006, para. 1).

First, this passage illustrates how commonly writers combine multiple modals to nuance the degree of certainty in their writing. Second, it shows us that modality is used on two levels: to project the writers' certainty about knowledge and to represent the certainty of other scholars who authored the knowledge. In the third sentence, the writers project moderate certainty by positioning the review as "recent" and acknowledging that "less is known" about this area, but they assign strong certainty to the authors of the review who "emphasized" the need for more research. Attributing strong certainty to these authors is a rhetorical move that helps make the argument for the writers' work. This same strategy is visible in the writers' use of strong modals such as "conclude", "cannot" and "no" in the final two sentences, marking the knowledge gap with confidence.

Finally, the way this passage opens deserves attention, because it raises the question, what is the 'right' degree of certainty to project? The opening sentence surprises us with its projection of weak certainty regarding the main problem statement, using the modal auxiliary "may be" and offering references to attribute the knowledge that medical students are stressed. The projection of uncertainty around this central claim makes us wonder, as readers, if there is some debate about the existence of stress in medical school. If so, this debate doesn't manifest in the rest of the paragraph. So perhaps it is just that the authors are performing an academic hedge, starting out with a cautious, uncertain tone as a way of conveying a neutral, 'scientific' stance as they open the paper. This sort of hedge can come across as insincere: we would prefer an unhedged opening sentence that claimed, as a matter of fact, that "To be a student in medical school is stressful."

This example raises the question: when is the academic hedge weakening your position as a writer rather than strengthening it? Getting modal "tuning" right is difficult, both for native English writers and for those writing in English as an additional language (EAL). One pattern of difficulty is that EAL writers may project stronger certainty than they intend, making 'categorical' assertions inappropriately (Yang et al. 2015). Another pattern of difficulty is that writers new to a scholarly conversation may project artificially weak degrees of certainty, as a way of managing the threat associated with wading into the scholarly fray. The next chapter will consider this situation in more detail. For now, our message is to be conscious and strategic about how you project certainty in your writing. Ask yourself, what do I think is true? What do my readers think? How can modality help me negotiate the relationship between those positions?

21.4   Conclusion

By wielding epistemic modal verbs and adverbs with skill, you can project degrees of certainty strategically and effectively in your writing. It is not a question of having "too much" or "too little" modality; scientific discourse is always modalized. The question is *how* you have modalized – how you have expressed your judgment about the degree of probability or factual status of the points in your argument -- and whether this modal tuning serves your rhetorical purposes.

See One, Do One, Teach One

1. Choose a paragraph from your paper. Underline all the epistemic modal verbs and adverbs you have used.
2. For each clause, assess where it sits on the epistemic modality spectrum: weak/speculative, intermediary/probabilitive, or strong/assertive.
3. Try tuning some of the sentences up or down by altering the verb or adverb.
4. Focus on your literature review: how have you used epistemic modality to map the known and the gap?

References

Chen, H. (2010). Contrastive learner corpus analysis of epistemic modality and interlanguage pragmatic competence in L2 writing. *Arizona Working Papers in SLA & Teaching, 17*, 27–51. https://journals.uair.arizona.edu/index.php/AZSLAT/article/view/21239

Hyland, K. (1996). Writing without conviction? Hedging in science research articles. *Applied Linguistics, 17*(4), 433–454. https://doi.org/10.1093/applin/17.4.433.

Hyland, K. (1998). Boosting, hedging and the negotiation of academic knowledge. *Talk and Text, 18*(3), 349–382.

Kjeldstadli, K., Tyssen, R., Finset, A., Hem, E., Gude, T., Gronvold, N. T., Ekeberg, O., et al. (2006). Life satisfaction and resilience in medical school – A six-year longitudinal, nationwide and comparative study. *BMC Medical Education, 6*, 48. https://doi.org/10.1186/1472-6920-6-48.

Myers, G. (1989). The pragmatics of politeness in scientific articles. *Applied Linguistics, 10*(1), 1–35. https://doi.org/10.1093/applin/10.1.1.

Yang, A., Zheng, S., & Ge, G. (2015). Epistemic modality in English-medium medical research articles: A systemic functional perspective. *English for Specific Purposes, 38*, 1–10. https://doi.org/10.1016/j.esp.2014.10.005.

Chapter 22
The Academic Hedge, Part II: Getting Politeness Right in Your Research Writing

> *The boldness of his mind was sheathed in a scabbard of politeness.*
>
> –Dumas Malone

Empirical research manuscripts rarely burn up the page. Letters to the editor sometimes do, and invited commentaries can, too. In these genres, even the customarily cautious academic writer can let her passions run away with her, issuing blistering judgments of others' work or preaching definitively from her high horse. But this doesn't happen very often. Research manuscripts tend to be more cautious than candid, more reserved than assertive. This flavor comes from epistemic modality, the linguistic means by which writers express their judgments about the degree of probability or factual status of a proposition.

Academic writers use epistemic modality in two ways. The first, described in the previous chapter, is to indicate the degree of certainty of a proposition and their confidence in it. The second is to negotiate a social interaction with the reader. This pragmatic function is critical in academic writing. Writing may not involve face-to-face contact, but it is nevertheless a form of social interaction; writers are joining a conversation among scholars in their field. This chapter offers strategies to help you participate in that conversation with the appropriate degree of politeness. Too little politeness and you can sound as though you don't recognize or respect the nuances of the scholarly conversation; too much and you can sound as though you have nothing substantive to add to it. Politeness is particularly necessary in three common rhetorical situations in your academic writing: denying other scholars' claims, making your own claims, and coining new terms. If you can get politeness right in these situations, readers are more likely to feel solidarity with you and to accept your contributions.

22.1   Politeness Theory

Joining a scholarly conversation means making a claim to knowledge. If you don't make a claim, you're not joining the conversation, you're just summarizing it. But making a claim always involves a tension: "the writer must stay within a certain consensus to have anything to say to members of his or her discipline, but must also have a new claim to make to justify publication" (Myers 1989, p. 5). This is a tricky rhetorical situation. Connecting insights from scholars of academic writing, Swales et al. (1998) explains that writers are in a "precarious relationship" with their readers because they must speak both as "humble servants" of their field and as "irreverent pioneers" forging beyond its established limits (p. 2). Politeness theory helps explain how writers successfully navigate this situation.

Politeness theory describes how speakers perform inter-personally sensitive communications in a nonthreatening or less threatening manner, in order to save their own "face" or that of their addressee (Brown and Levinson 1987). Face refers to the public self-image that individuals endeavor to protect. Linguists distinguish between positive and negative politeness, depending on the type of face that is being maintained or threatened. Positive face involves a desire for connection with others and refers to one's self-esteem, while negative face needs include autonomy and independence, one's freedom to act (Brown and Levinson 1987). During any social interaction, participants cooperate to maintain these aspects of one another's face.

Even apparently mundane communication can constitute a face-threatening act (FTA), depending on the social distance between speaker and addressee. For instance, say you are ready to review a draft research paper being produced by a colleague and you would like it sent asap, while your time is available. You can make this request in a number of ways. You could say:

Send the draft for review.
Please send the draft for review.
Would you mind sending the draft for review?
I've had a meeting cancelled, so I have time to review your draft.

The first option commits the FTA baldly, without redress and there are few situations in which this would not sound abrupt. Each subsequent option introduces more politeness to redress the FTA presented by your request. How much politeness you choose to use depends on your relationship with the writer. If you are talking to colleague you've known for years, "Please send the draft for review" is likely sufficient. "Please could you ..." uses the conditional to lessen the FTA even more; perhaps if you're asking for the second or third time, you might feel the need to "turn up" the politeness in this manner. However, if you're talking to your Dean, you might choose the last option, which describes your availability, rather than making the request directly. This is described as doing the FTA off the record, by implication. In choosing this option, you redress both the threat to your Dean's negative face (her freedom to do as she wishes) and the threat to your own positive face (your desire to avoid the embarrassment of refusal). As these examples show, the FTA presented by a request is always influenced by power relations, social distance and, therefore, the degree of imposition it constitutes (Brown and Levinson 1987).

22.2 Politeness Strategies in Scientific Writing

What has politeness theory to do with writing a health research paper? First, it offers a language to talk about the academic hedge – those rhetorical moves of caution, uncertainty and deference that writers make. Second, it helps you to judge when you should adopt the same moves. Because if you simply offer your criticisms of existing knowledge, your study findings, or your erudite conclusions as efficiently and clearly as possible, you will not be cooperating to save face – yours, your fellow researchers', or your readers'.

Any new claim to knowledge a writer makes in a scientific article constitutes a face-threatening act. Myers (1989) argues that the weight of that FTA is "related to the size of the claim and the number of researchers who would have to alter their practices if it were accepted" (p. 5). The weightier the face-threatening act, the more politeness will be used to redress it. Take the following example:

> It has become apparent to many that something is amiss with the practice of research in the medical education field, and several of our key leaders have expressed concerns. However, we seem to still be struggling to identify exactly what the problem is. We have scientific models of research to emulate, but, despite our efforts to follow these models, we are not sure that we are getting where we want to go, and we are not sure where we are going wrong. (Regehr 2010, p. 44)

This comes from the introduction of a paper that challenges the fundamental metaphor underlying medical education. To mitigate the FTA associated with this powerful claim, Regehr (2010) employs layers of epistemic modality and politeness. Expressions of epistemic modality-- "it has become apparent", "something is amiss with", "seem to still be struggling", and "are not sure" – create a tone of speculation, a hedge against readers disagreeing with the strong position the paper takes. In addition, the use of inclusive pronouns such as "we" and "our" allows Regehr (2010) to invoke the discipline as a whole and thus include himself in those who are "struggling" and "going wrong".

Even if the claim you wish to make in your writing does not seem (to you) to be profoundly threatening to conventional knowledge in your field, you may still need to employ politeness strategies to hedge it. In appreciating how to use politeness and hedging in your own academic writing, Myers' (1989) description of three recurring rhetorical situations can be helpful: denying a claim, making a claim, and coining new terms.

22.2.1   *Denying a Claim*

Setting up the problem space for your paper requires a critical summary of the limits of existing knowledge. Myers (1989) calls this 'denying a claim', and it constitutes a FTA not only for the reader but also for the writer. Novice writers can feel this threat with particular acuteness, wondering 'who am I to critique the eminent scholars I've read?' One way to mitigate the FTA in this situation is to depersonalize it, using pronouns that include the writer in the criticism and create solidarity with readers, as illustrated in the example above.

Depersonalizing, like all epistemic modality, is a matter of degree, and learning to tune it up or down can help you participate purposefully within the social interaction of scholarship. Consider the depersonalizing strategies in the following example, which we have bolded:

> **Many scholars believe** a focus on outcomes promises to produce better doctors and mitigate challenges faced in the evolving health care landscape.[6][29] Although **its conceptual basis may make intuitive sense, concerns have been raised** about the paucity of empirical evidence[4, 10, 11] supporting the competency-based approach and the 'revolutionary rhetoric' used to promote it.[12] Further, **some researchers question** the theoretical underpinnings of the model,[13][15][16] as well as the feasibility of its practical application in medicine.[11, 17] Within the academic literature, **instrumental arguments for and against CBME are well established.** (Boyd et al. 2018, p. 45)

This passage presents what linguists would call a "denial" of CBME's claims, hedged for politeness through a number of depersonalizing strategies. These include use of third person rather than author names to avoid direct attribution ("Many scholars", "some researchers"), positioning things rather than people as the subject ("its conceptual basis"), and employing passive voice to remove the agent of the verb altogether ("have been raised", "are well established").

This example also shows that politeness need not produce mincing prose or a weak authorial stance: you can hold a strong position as a writer and still invoke politeness strategies. Boyd et al. (2018) achieve this by counterbalancing depersonalizing strategies with verb choices (underlined in the passage) that intensify rather than mitigate their face-threatening act of denying CBME's claims. In a literature review, writers position themselves and other scholars in the field as either affiliated with, or distanced from one another's knowledge claims, and verbs are a strong signal of this evaluative positioning (see Chap. 4). Boyd et al. (2018) distance themselves from the many scholars who "believe" in and "promote" the outcomes focus, because both verbs connote unscientific stances. Intuition is similarly problematic in scientific thinking; thus, the statement that the concept of CBME "may make intuitive sense" not only signals divisions in the scholarly community but also positions the authors on one side of that divide.

22.2.2   *Making a Claim*

Just as denying a claim is a face-threatening act, so too is making a claim. A common form of politeness for a statement of a claim is to attribute it to some impersonal agency (Brown and Levinson 1987), by using language such as "this finding suggests", "as this example illustrates", "these observations demonstrate", or by employing the passive voice to remove the agent from the sentence altogether. In the following example, Varpio et al. (2017) employ a number of these impersonalizing strategies (which we have bolded) to redress the threat as they mount the central claim of their paper:

> **This is an example** of the 'cobra effect'[1] (i.e. the unintended consequence) that we, as qualitative researchers, have helped to create: **the strategies** that helped to legitimise qualitative research **have not been sufficiently discussed and examined** in the HPE literature and so, **left** un-problematised, **they are often adopted** as a set of standards that should be applied to all qualitative research. (p. 41)

In this passage, "the strategies" have agency rather than researchers using the strategies, and many of the verbs are in the passive voice: "have not been sufficiently discussed and examined", "left" and "are often adopted". You know that you have come across the passive voice when you are inclined to ask, "by whom?" Here, passive voice reduces the threat to the face of qualitative researchers by removing them as explicit agents.

This impersonal nature of much academic writing should not be read as a reflection of the neutrality or objectivity of science – in fact, Myers (1989) argues, quite the opposite. It is a manifestation of writers dealing with the social implications of their knowledge claims within a scholarly community (Swales et al. 1998). This is demonstrated in the Varpio et al. (2017) example, where the authors' use of impersonalizing devices is combined with the use of an inclusive pronoun. Demonstrating that they are aware that their thesis represents a FTA for others in the qualitative research community, they acknowledge that, "we, as qualitative researchers, have helped to create" the problem exposed in the paper.

Hedging is another way to introduce politeness when making a claim. Hedging abounds in academic writing, marking the writer's claims as provisional, pending community acceptance. Hedges allow writers to imply that "a statement is based on plausible reasoning rather than certain knowledge, and allow readers the freedom to dispute it" (Hyland 1998, p 353). Many common phrases are hedges: for instance, "to our knowledge" is a hedge against the possibility that the writers' knowledge might be incomplete; "our findings suggest" or "we believe" is a hedge against researcher misinterpretation or contradiction by others' findings; and "seem to be" is a hedge against the possibility that appearances may be deceiving.

Hedging is an important convention in the research manuscript genre because it offers a resource for writers to express their claims with "precision, caution, and modesty" (Hyland 1996, p. 251). It is particularly prominent in the introduction section when the writer initially presents their claim(s), as examples earlier in this paper have illustrated, and in the Discussion and Conclusion sections where the

Table 22.1 Four grammatical techniques for hedging

Modal verb	If…then	Modifier (adverb or adjective)	Implying alternatives
"The argument would hold that…"	"If this conclusion is sound, then …"	"Only 2 studies suggest…"	"One theory proposes that…"
"Professional identity could be understood as…"	"If this argument holds, then …"	"We can only speculate …"	"Lawson offers a model for…"
"This may provide evidence that…"	"If these findings are sound, then…"	"Arguably, survey research represents a population…"	"An implication of this finding is …"
		"Possibly, role modelling has been misunderstood …"	

writer offers implications for consideration by the scholarly community. Consider these examples, with hedges bolded, from the opening paragraphs of a Discussion section (Choudhury and Asan 2020):

> "**To our knowledge**, this is the first systematic review exploring and portraying studies that show the influence of AI (machine-learning and natural language processing techniques) on clinical-level patient safety outcomes."
>
> "**Despite** varying AI performance, **most** studies have reported a positive impact on safety outcomes (Table 2), thus indicating that safety outcomes do not **necessarily** correlate to AI performance measures [26]."
>
> "**According to our review**, AI algorithms are **rarely** scrutinized against a standard of care (clinicians or clinical gold standard)."
>
> "Relying on AI outcomes that have not been evaluated against a standard benchmark that meets clinical requirements **can be** misleading."

These examples also use depersonalization through third person ("studies" are the agents rather than researchers who conduct them) and passive voice ("are rarely scrutinized" "have not been evaluating against"), as a way of infusing politeness while making claims.

Grammatically, hedging is done in a number of ways: with a modal verb making a conditional statement (e.g., "would", "could", "can"); with an "if … then" conditional construction; with a modifier (e.g., "probably", "possibly", "likely", "rarely"); or with any device suggesting alternatives or exceptions (e.g., use of indefinite rather than definite articles: "a" conclusion, not "the" conclusion). Table 22.1 illustrates how these four options are constructed.

22.2.3 Coining New Terms

As Myers (1989) cautions: "to offer a new term for a phenomenon … is to invite the question, 'Who are *you* to name this stuff?'" (p. 6) Introducing new terms is threatening; it both constrains the freedom of the reader and exposes the writer to the possibility of the community's rejection. Therefore, the introduction of a new term will use hedging to mark its provisional nature; as the term becomes accepted, hedging of its use will recede.

As an example, consider the evolution of hedging associated with the term "collective competence" which Lorelei introduced to the field of health professions education. Her introduction of the term signalled its provisionality subject to community adoption: she suggested that "the emergence of what I will call a 'collectivist discourse of competence' reflects growing attention in the social and organizational spheres to healthcare's nature as a complex system. 'Collective competence' draws on social learning theory" (Lingard 2009, p. 626). In keeping with Myers' (1989) point that any reference to a person dilutes the FTA of a claim, she referred to herself in introducing this new term ("what I will call a collectivist discourse"). Further, by using quotation marks around the term "collective competence", she marked its status as speculation, not accepted knowledge. As the years go by, Lorelei has gradually used the term without explicitly invoking herself as the person behind it or putting it in quotation marks, but the provisional flavor remains, achieved by using a reference to locate and attribute the term, as in this 2016 paper: "In fact, we can explain these paradoxical truths only by reference to collective competence. Collective competence is a distributed capacity of a system, not easily reducible to an individual; it is dynamic and strongly tied to context." (Lingard 2016, p. S20).

In 2018, Lorelei was getting a bit frustrated that the assessment literature had largely ignored the concept in the ten years since she introduced it. She threatened her own face by acknowledging that situation: "The concept of collective competence entered medical education discourse in 2008; however, our field has yet to find a meaningful way to translate this into assessment practices" (Sebok-Syer et al. 2018, p. 978). However, this threat to her face was counterbalanced by three other features in the sentence. First, in using "the concept of collective competence" as the agent of the verb "entered", she presented the concept as being ignored, not herself. Second, in using "our field" she included herself in those who are struggling to translate the concept. Third, with the construction "has yet to find a meaningful way to translate this", she introduced the hedge that this is a temporary situation.

Hedging is a complex dance. It is a matter of degrees; therefore, writers can be insufficiently or overly polite in their research writing. Too little politeness and the writer may appear to be either naively treating knowledge as a set of disembodied facts or making categorical assertions that are unwarranted. Too much politeness and the writer might struggle to demonstrate control of the scholarly conversation and a critical position within it.

Hedging is not just about degrees, it is also about context. Hedge when you mean it, not simply to perform academic obeisance to a senior colleague. You can come across as insincere if you hedge in the wrong moments, such as hedges that function as back-handed compliments:

Although perhaps the most influential in the field to date, Levac's work overlooks the question of gender.

Hedging that is out of proportion can also appear more face-threatening than it otherwise would (Ginsburg et al. 2015). Consider the following two examples:

If the idea of collective competence is embraced, **then** it **could** call into question the foundation of assessment during clinical training.

The idea of collective competence **could** call into question the foundation of assessment during clinical training.

Both sentences use "could" to hedge, to weaken the suggestion being made by the writer. But the first example also uses an "If . . . then" conditional construction which intensifies the hedge, increases the FTA.

You can also appear self contradictory if you hedge carelessly. Consider this hedge that expresses tentativeness, only to immediately refute that stance with a bald assertion:

Medical educators have **recently begun to wonder whether and how** incivility in the clinical workplace **might** impact trainees. Incivility is rampant and destructive in many training contexts.

These two sentences are jarring in juxtaposition, because the first is extensively hedged and the second is not hedged at all. If the juxtaposition is the point – that is, if the writer wishes to call out the tentativeness of medical educators 'wondering' as an epidemic of incivility rages – then adding a *booster* to the second sentence would make this more clear: "Incivility, *in fact* (or *of course*, or *as we know*) is rampant and destructive . . . . ".

Finally, do not mistake hedging for insipid, mealy-mouthed discourse. As the examples above illustrate, authors who hedge can occupy strong rhetorical positions, critique dominant ideas and provoke impassioned reader responses (Norman 2011; Regehr 2011). They *can* burn up the page. Ideally, though, hedging allows them to do so in ways that spark constructive debate rather than unintended offense.

22.3 Conclusion

Because publishing your research is a social act, you must carefully attend to the relationships you construct between yourself, your readers, and your colleagues in the scholarly community. The academic hedge, achieved through politeness strategies, allows you to stress solidarity with your readers, evaluate the state of knowledge in the field, project humility and respect as you make even strong claims, and cooperate in the social act of advancing knowledge.

See One, Do One, Teach One
1. Assess the hedge
   Reread your literature review. Flag any sentence where you have referenced an existing knowledge claim. This is a potentially face-threatening act, particularly if you are denying the claim. Now, assess how (whether?) you have used hedging to mitigate that threat. Refer back

(continued)

to Table 22.1 and identify features such as modal verbs, modifiers, if...then constructions, and implying alternatives. Check whether you have employed depersonalizing strategies such as passive voice or inclusive 'we' statements.

2. Have you been a bit aggressive? Try to strengthen the hedge:

   (a) Increase the depersonalization (e.g., change active to passive voice).
   (b) Try using modal verbs (e.g., could, may, might)

3. Have you been too tentative? Try to weaken the hedge:

   (a) Change conditional constructions to declarative statements
   (b) Check your adverbs and adjectives. If they inject uncertainty (e.g., possibly), remove them or change them (e.g., invariably).

   Repeat this exercise for your Results and Discussion sections to assess your use of hedging when you are making a claim or coining new language.

   Sometimes it is easier to 'feel' politeness at work in writing when it's not your own draft. Trade drafts with a colleague and review a selected section for hedging using the above questions to guide you. This can be a useful way to get focused reader feedback if you're concerned about wading into an established scholarly conversation and getting the tone right.

References

Boyd, V. A., Whitehead, C. R., Thille, P., Ginsburg, S., Brydges, R., & Kuper, A. (2018). Competency-based medical education: The discourse of infallibility. *Medical Education, 52* (1), 45–57. https://doi.org/10.1111/medu.13467.

Brown, P., & Levinson, S. C. (1987). *Politeness: Some universals in language usage.* London: Cambridge University Press.

Choudhury, A., & Asan, O. (2020). Role of artificial intelligence in patient safety outcomes: Systematic literature review. *JMIR Medical Informatics, 8*(7), e18599.

Ginsburg, S., Van der Vleuten, C., Eva, K., & Lingard, L. (2015). Hedging to save face: A linguistic analysis of written comments on in-training evaluation reports. *Advances in Health Sciences Education, 21*, 175–188. https://doi.org/10.1007/s10459-015-9622-0.

Hyland, K. (1996). Talking to the academy: Forms of hedging in science research articles. *Written Communication, 13*(2), 251–281. https://doi.org/10.1177/0741088396013002004.

Hyland, K. (1998). Boosting, hedging and the negotiation of academic knowledge. *Talk and Text, 18*(3), 349–382.

Lingard, L. (2009). What we see and don't see when we look at 'competence': Notes on a god term. *Advances in Health Sciences Education, 14*(5), 625–628. https://doi.org/10.1007/s10459-009-9206-y.

Lingard, L. (2016). Paradoxical truths and persistent myths: Reframing the team competence conversation. *Journal of Continuing Education in the Health Professions, 36*, S19–S21. https://doi.org/10.1097/CEH.0000000000000078.

Malone, D. (1948). Jefferson the Virginian. In *Jefferson and his time* (Vol. 1). Charlottesville: First University of Virginia Press.

Myers, G. (1989). The pragmatics of politeness in scientific articles. *Applied Linguistics, 10*(1), 35. https://doi.org/10.1093/applin/10.1.1.

Norman, G. (2011). Chaos, complexity and complicatedness: Lessons from rocket science. *Medical Education, 45*(6), 549–559. https://doi.org/10.1111/j.1365-2923.2011.03945.x.

Regehr, G. (2010). It's NOT rocket science: Rethinking our metaphors for research in health professions education. *Medical Education, 44*(1), 31–39. https://doi.org/10.1111/j.1365-2923.2009.03418.x.

Regehr, G. (2011). Highway spotters and traffic controllers: Further reflections on complexity. *Medical Education, 45*(6), 542–543. https://doi.org/10.1111/j.1365-2923.2011.04007.x.

Sebok-Syer, S., Chahine, S., Watling, C. J., Goldszmidt, M., Cristancho, S., & Lingard, L. (2018). Considering the interdependence of clinical performance: Implications for assessment and entrustment. *Medical Education, 52*(9), 970–980. https://doi.org/10.1111/medu.13588.

Swales, J. M., Ahmad, U., Chang, Y., Chavez, D., Dressen, D. F., & Seymour, R. (1998). Consider this: The role of imperatives in scholarly writing. *Applied Linguistics, 19*(1), 97–121. https://doi.org/10.1093/applin/19.1.97.

Varpio, L., Ajjawi, R., Monrouxe, L. V., O'Brien, B. C., & Rees, C. E. (2017). Shedding the cobra effect: Problematising thematic emergence, triangulation, saturation and member checking. *Medical Education, 51*(1), 40–50. https://doi.org/10.1111/medu.13124.

Chapter 23
From Silent to Audible Voice: Adjusting Register, Stance & Engagement in Your Writing

We recently asked a group of doctoral candidates in a writing workshop, "What kind of voice do you want to have in your writing?" "Clear" and "logical" were popular answers, but not exactly what we were getting at. Then a young woman put up her hand and announced, "I want to be a courageous writer". Wow, okay. So how do we achieve that? What would a courageous scientific voice sound like, exactly, and which features would we play with to make such a voice apparent and acceptable? In this chapter, we explore strategies for identifying and creating voice in scientific writing.

Voice "creates the illusion that the writer is speaking directly to the reader from the page" (Clark 2006, p. 105). For poets, novelists, journalists, songwriters, play-wrights, and screenwriters, voice is everything – their success depends on establishing a voice that is distinct and recognizable. For academic writers, too, a recognizable voice brings credibility to the writing. But establishing a distinctive voice can be challenging. For one thing, authorship is typically shared; writing as "we" rather than as "I" may stifle an individual's voice. For another, the genres in which we write can confine us, seeming to leave little room for unique voices.

Let's consider the expectations of the academic world: what are scientific writers supposed to sound like? Science has conventionally required a distant, formal, impersonal – one might even say 'silent' –authorial voice. Originating in the natural sciences, this expectation has found its way into the health and social sciences through the IMRD genre with its positivist underpinnings. Positivism posits that knowledge is 'out there', potentially discoverable by anyone properly trained to unearth it. Findings, therefore, are separate from the researcher, justifying a distant, impersonal authorial voice (Gray 2017). This authorial voice is not just a matter of rhetorical technique, however; it is also a matter of symbolic power. Why? Because "silent authorship comes to mark mature scholarship", and eventually the "proper voice is no voice at all" (Charmaz and Mitchell 1996, p 286). Thus authors taking up the IMRD genre are socialized into silence: "to keep their voices out of the reports they produce, to emulate Victorian children: be seen (in the credits) not heard

L. Lingard, C. Watling, *Story, Not Study: 30 Brief Lessons to Inspire Health Researchers as Writers*, Innovation and Change in Professional Education 19, https://doi.org/10.1007/978-3-030-71363-8_23

(in the text)" (Charmaz and Mitchell 1996, p 285). Such socialization has powerful implications: for instance, nursing scholars have argued that the conventions of voice limit the ability of nursing researchers to reflect the humanity of their profession and to produce writing that is accessible to patients and practicing nurses (Mitchell 2017).

23.1   Challenging Conventions

The scientific manuscript has been called an "uptight genre", unreceptive to innovation (Hundt and Mair 1999). But the times, they are a-changing. Major philosophical shifts in science are creating fault lines in the conventions of scientific voice (Gray 2017). Traditional positivist assumptions have come under fire by constructivist theory and postmodernism, leading to a critique of researchers' representational authority (Gray 2017). The "facts" are no longer seen to speak for themselves in many health research fields, and the uncritical adoption of a traditional authorial voice is increasingly unacceptable (Charmaz and Mitchell 1996). Furthermore, longstanding habits (which many writers have taken to be rules) such as avoiding personal pronouns are falling out of favor: Sword's (2012) analysis of 500 research articles and 100 advanced academic writing guides concluded that the vast majority advocate "I" and "We". Change, however, is nonlinear and fluid: in 2020 one of us has been asked by a journal editor to replace "We" with "The authors" in the Methods section of an accepted empirical, qualitative paper.

   Authorial voice is also shifting as concerns emerge about the inaccessibility of published science and its failure to impact knowledge and behavior in the wider world. Some fear that "the science community will lose its voice, drowned out by either the new anti-science movement or just the cacophony of society's noise" (Olson 2009, p. 8).There are increasing calls for science writers to become better storytellers, to speak more directly and engagingly to readers, both their research peers and the lay public (Hunter 2016). However, while some powerful examples exist (think Carl Sagan or Oliver Sacks), resistance to change is powerful. One of us, after consciously aiming for a more engaging authorial voice, was told by an associate editor that they "prefer a less dramatic style of writing"; the other had a reviewer express discomfort that "formal academic writing conventions were stretched" in a manuscript, largely because of the use of uncommon but evocative verbs. An "uptight" genre indeed!

   How, then, should a writer determine the right authorial voice for her paper? How formal should it be? How specialized? How impersonal? And, if you're trying something a bit outside the convention, how can you strategically increase your chances of success? Next, we describe how writers can play with three dimensions -- register, stance and engagement – to find a voice that will be both compelling and acceptable to reviewers and readers.

23.2   Register

Register is the level of formality of the language you use. Five registers exist. From most to least formal they are: frozen, formal, consultative, casual, and intimate. Science communication commonly dwells in the 'formal' register, but also has aspects which are 'frozen', such as the informed consent template in a research ethics application. Register is achieved through vocabulary, punctuation, and grammatical features. These are illustrated in Table 23.1.

Consider how the following examples employ these features to change the register of this sentence, making it increasingly informal.

Questions have been raised regarding the impact of root cause analysis (RCA) on patient safety.
We question the impact of root cause analysis (RCA) on patient safety.
To what extent does root cause analysis (RCA) impact patient safety?
Does an analysis of what causes an error *really* impact patient safety?

The first sentence is the most formal due to the combination of specialized terms (RCA), full verb constructions, indirect construction of a question, third person point of view and passive voice (have been raised). The second sentence retains the specialized term (RCA) but shifts to first person point of view (We) and active voice (question).The third sentence asks a direct question, which increases informality, but the phrase "to what extent" is a prose feature that retains some formality. The fourth sentence removes this expression, increasing the directness of the question; it also adds a colloquial adverb (really) and, for more informality, uses italics to emphasize it.

Choosing a register requires careful thought about audience. The right register for one audience could very well be the wrong one for another. Take this chapter, for

Table 23.1 Features of register

Vocabulary		Punctuation		Grammar	
Formal	Informal	Formal	Informal	Formal	Informal
Specialized terms	Slang, plain language	Full verb constructions	Contractions	Complex sentences	Simple sentences
Latin or other foreign expressions	Standard English	Punctuation for accuracy rather than mood	Exclamation & question marks; italics & dashes for emphasis	Indirect constructions (conditionals, implied questions)	Direct questions
Prose features (things you write but don't say, like 'insofar as')	Speech features, colloquialisms	Complete words	Abbreviations	Passive voice	Active voice
				3rd person point of view	1st and 2nd person point of view

instance. Our goal is to translate highly specialized linguistic knowledge to a health research audience; therefore, we are converting jargon to plain language, writing in simple rather than complex sentences, being explicit and direct rather than implying. We've chosen clarity and accessibility over nuance in some places. And, while we keep envisioning a cringing linguist reading this, we have reconciled ourselves to the idea that if we get register right for our target audience, the cringing linguist is likely to be appalled but sympathetic.

23.3   Stance

In scientific writing, the intended reader is part of the ongoing scholarly conversation, and they can always refute the writer's claims. Therefore, writers must carefully situate themselves, anticipating and engaging with their readers' responses.

Writers express a persona that their readers can recognize and respect. Hyland (2005) calls this "stance", which is made up of three elements: evidentiality, affect, and presence. Evidentiality illustrates the writer's degree of commitment to what they're saying, through hedges and boosters; affect signals the writer's attitudes and emotions about what they're saying; and presence is the extent to which the writer refers to herself in the text (Hyland 2005). Table 23.2 defines and illustrates the grammatical features that accomplish each component.

As the two examples in Table 23.2 illustrate, stance differs according to both genre and discipline. The commentary has more pronounced affect, while the empirical research paper is more analytical than evocative. This pattern is shifting, however, particularly in qualitative social sciences which value the subjectivity of the researcher. Ethnographers, for instance, have argued for more evocative empirical writing, asserting that "we do ourselves and our disciplines no service by ... suppressing wonder or perplexity or dread" (Mitchell 2017, p. 300). Evidentiality is prominent in both the examples due to their academic context, but boosters sit more comfortably in a commentary where writers tend to take a stronger position than in empirical papers, which hedge to acknowledge complexity and debate. Self mention can be found in both genres, but more commonly empirical research papers efface the author through the passive voice.

Corpus analysis research also describes disciplinary differences in stance. For instance, writers in the natural sciences use fewer boosters, attitude markers, and self mentions than in the social sciences (Charles 2006; Seoane and Hundt 2018). This makes sense as it reflects the dominant epistemology of these disciplines. Natural sciences are objectivist: procedures matter, not researchers. Social sciences are interpretivist: researchers *are* the procedures in many cases. Given that health research often sits between these disciplinary positions and shares values with both of them, we advise writers to listen for the type and frequency of stance markers that are customary in their health research field.

Table 23.2 Features of stance

Grammar Feature	Evidentiality		Affect	Presence
	Hedges	Boosters	Attitude markers	Self mention
Purpose	Withhold complete commitment.	Express certainty.	Convey emotion and perspective.	Highlight the researcher role.
	Open space for dispute.	Establish solidarity with audience.	Assume and foster shared attitude in audience.	Acknowledge subjectivity. Invoke ethos.
Tools	Modal verbs (might, could) and modifiers (adverbs: perhaps, purportedly; adjectives: preliminary, possible)	Action verbs (demonstrate, assert, conclude) and modal adverbs (certainly, clearly, of course, highly)	Attitude verbs (prefer, believe); sentence adverbs (unfortunately) and adjectives (remarkable, challenging)	First person pronouns (I, we); possessive adjectives (my, our)
Examples: Commentary (Urbach et al. 2019)	"The evidence *suggests* so—but it takes time for population level implementation . . ."	"The checklist was *intentionally* designed as a tool to strengthen team communication, and these data suggest that *it does precisely this.*"	"Checklists, after all, are credited with *truly extraordinary* power, bordering on the *miraculous.*"	"*We* do not disagree."
Examples: Empirical research (Panda et al. 2020)	"These types of recovery data *could be shared* with family members or caregivers to promote engagement . . . ."	"*This is especially true* for patients with cancer, for whom multidisciplinary treatment makes it difficult to appreciate . . . ."	"This is *especially valuable* in fields . . . where the multidisciplinary management of cancer makes describing the physical outcomes . . . *challenging* for clinicians."	"*Our research group* continues to enroll patients from multiple surgical centers . . . ."

23.4 Engagement

Writers not only project themselves into their texts; they also project their readers. Engagement strategies allow writers to recognize the reader's presence, acknowledge their expectations, focus their attention, address their concerns, and guide their interpretation. Through engagement, readers are constructed as participants in the argument, with the ultimate rhetorical goal of soliciting their agreement. Hyland (2005) describes five main elements of engagement: reader pronouns, personal asides, appeals to shared knowledge, directives and questions. The purpose and grammatical features of each are described in Table 23.3.

A common engagement device in academic writing is the inclusive "we", which binds writer and reader together in attitude and argument: "We face a critical challenge in hospital management." This is distinct from the researchers-as-We,

Table 23.3 Features of engagement

	Reader pronouns	Personal asides	Appeals to shared knowledge	Directives	Questions
Purpose	Bind writer and reader	Interrupt to comment.	Establish, by presupposing, familiar or accepted knowledge	Direct reader interpretations or actions	Involve reader in discovery
		Create a sense of dialogue			
Grammatical features	Pronouns (You, your, We)	Brackets, dashes	Adverbs (of course, clearly, obviously).	Imperative verbs (*consider, note, see*).	Question terms (who, what, why, where, how, when)
	Possessives: (Our field; our community)		Propositions (it is understood, it is true, it is necessary that).	Modals of obligation (*must, should*).	Punctuation (?)
				Judgments (*It is important, it is essential*).	

which abounds in health research writing: e.g., "We were guided by three research questions." By contrast, "you" and "your" are rarely used to engage the academic reader, particularly in natural and medical sciences. An exception is methodological guides, which may use the second person to address the reader directly. For example:

You can develop your own voice by experimenting with word choice and sentence length.

Our use of second person in this book is a way of speaking directly to you as a reader - an effort to create the impression of a guide or coach looking over your shoulder The second person can come across as 'preachy', though, so we combine it with politeness markers and self-critique to hopefully minimize preaching and maximize conversation.

Personal asides allow the writer to step away from line of argument, to reflect, to detour, to whisper in the reader's ear. They are usually signalled by brackets or dashes. For instance, you might write:

Notwithstanding the different (and to some extent incommensurable) perspectives represented by the above literature . . .

This aside engages the reader in noting the "incommensurable" nature of perspectives without the writer needing to evidence or elaborate that claim. Discursive footnotes, in the journals that allow them, can also serve this function.

Appeals to shared knowledge position the reader as agreeing with certain premises. Consider this example: "It is a truth universally acknowledged by policymakers, researchers and research funding bodies that patients and the public should be 'involved' in research . . ." (Greenhalgh 2009 p. 338). Hyland (2005) notes that writers can use this strategy either to ask readers to recognize familiar ideas, or "to smuggle contested ideas into their argument" (184). The preceding example is not smuggling: "truth universally acknowledged" is too strong an assertion for any sleight of hand. (And the Jane Austen allusion likely reverbates, feeling familiar even if readers can't quite discern why.) But consider this example:

> Given the increasing value of qualitative methods in health research, it is crucial that review criteria are refined and expanded to include qualitative standards.

This sentence presents as a "given" the value of qualitative methods in health research, in order to argue for changes to journal review criteria. However, those defending traditional review criteria are likely to view the "value of qualitative methods" as a contested idea. Tucked into the subordinate clause, however, it appears as a shared premise rather than one open to debate.

Directives instruct the reader to perform an action or to see an issue in a way determined by the writer. Of the types of directives that Hyland (2005) enumerates, two are most relevant here. Textual directives steer readers from one part of the text to another: e.g., "See Appendix 1 for a full accounting of our search strategy." Cognitive directives guide readers through a line of reasoning, or encourage them to take a particular stance:

> Therefore, as we trace the construction and use of discourses within the CBME literature, the reader must remember that particular ways of thinking or writing are not necessarily conscious or deliberate" (Boyd et al. 2018, p. 47).

This is a very assertive directive, explicitly invoking "the reader" and using an imperative verb "must remember".

Questions present an unresolved issue and encourage the reader to share the writer's curiosity. They can create the sense that writer and reader are discovering the answer together. However, a corpus analysis of research articles from eight disciplines found that most questions are rhetorical: the reader appears to be the judge, but the writer is in charge. This is particularly the case when a question posed is followed immediately by its answer:

> How might this model of 'comfort with uncertainty' inform how educators support the development of clinical reasoning in trainees? We offer three preliminary educational implications that follow from this exploration of 'comfort with uncertainty.' First, ... (Ilgen et al. 2019, p. 804)

With engagement strategies, a little goes a long way. One or two questions work beautifully; ten fall flat. Overused brackets can feel meandering, undermining your logic. Multiple directives can feel gimmicky, like breaking the fourth wall in film. Be selective about which engagement strategies you employ, and use them sparingly.

23.5 Conclusion

Voice is not accidental; it reflects deliberate authorial choices. Learning to analyze writing – both your own and others' – helps to bring these choices to conscious awareness. If your go-to voice is silent, distant and impersonal, consider what you might achieve by playing with that a little bit. Of course, you must consider disciplinary conventions and journal expectations, but don't be hemmed in by out-of-date assumptions about what is "allowed". Try shifting where you situate on the continuum between personal and impersonal, close and distant, general and special-ized, subjective and objective, evocative and analytical. Remember that your voice can change over the course of a manuscript: perhaps an impersonal and analytical Methods section told in the third person with specialized terminology and passive voice, and a more personal, interactive Implications section with first person, direct questions, and appeals to shared knowledge. Be courageous – go out on a limb and try something provocative. Get feedback from thoughtful readers to see what worked and, yes, what didn't. But make your voice heard.

See One, Do One, Teach One
1. Using Table 23.1 as a guide, assess your register in your manuscript.

   (a) How formal or informal are you? Does your register change in places? Is that purposeful and effective?
   (b) Play with your register by altering vocabulary, punctuation or grammar.

2. Using Table 23.2 as a guide, assess your stance in the manuscript.

   (a) Are you close or distant? Personal or impersonal? Might it work to have a more personal stance in the 'story' sections of the manuscript (Intro and Discussion), more impersonal in the 'study' (Methods and Results) sections?
   (b) Try shifting your stance by altering evidentiality, affect or presence.

3. Using Table 23.3 as a guide, assess how you have engaged with your reader.

   (a) How have you constructed your reader?
   (b) Alter your engagement by playing with reader pronouns, personal asides, appeals to shared knowledge, directives, and questions.

References

Boyd, V. A., Whitehead, C. R., Thille, P., Ginsburg, S., Brydges, R., & Kuper, A. (2018). Competency-based medical education: The discourse of infallibility. *Medical Education, 52* (1), 45–57. https://doi.org/10.1111/medu.13467.
Charles, M. (2006). The construction of stance in reporting clauses: A cross-disciplinary study of theses. *Applied Linguistics, 27*(3), 492–518. https://doi.org/10.1093/applin/aml021.
Charmaz, K., & Mitchell, R. G. (1996). The myth of silent authorship: Self, substance, and style in ethnographic writing. *Symbolic Interaction, 19*(4), 285–302. https://doi.org/10.1525/si.1996.19. 4.285.
Clark, R. P. (2006). *Writing tools.* New York: Little, Brown, and Company.
Gray, G. (2017). Academic voice in scholarly writing. *The Qualitative Report, 22*(1), 179–196. https://nsuworks.nova.edu/tqr/vol22/iss1/10.

Greenhalgh, P. (2009). Patient and public involvement in chronic illness: Beyond the expert patient. *BMJ, 338*, b49. https://doi.org/10.1136/bmj.b49.

Hundt, M., & Mair, C. (1999). Agile and uptight genres: The corpus-based approach to language change in progress. *International Journal of Corpus Linguistics, 4*(2), 221–242. https://doi.org/10.1075/ijcl.4.2.02hun.

Hunter, P. (2016). The communications gap between scientists and public. *Science & Society EMBO Reports, 17*(11), 1513–1515. https://doi.org/10.15252/embr.201643379.

Hyland, K. (2005). Stance and engagement: A model of interaction in academic discourse. *Discourse Studies, 7*(2), 173–192. https://doi.org/10.1177/1461445605050365.

Ilgen, J., Eva, K., de Bruin, A., Cook, D., & Regehr, G. (2019). Comfort with uncertainty: Reframing our conceptions of how clinicians navigate complex clinical situations. *Advances in Health Sciences Education, 24*(4), 797–809. https://doi.org/10.1007/s10459-018-9859-5.

Mitchell, K. M. (2017). Academic voice: On feminism, presence, and objectivity in writing. *Nursing Inquiry, 24*(4). https://doi.org/10.1111/nin.12200.

Olson, R. (2009). *Don't be such a scientist: Talking substance in an age of style*. Washington, DC: Island Press.

Panda, N., Solsky, I., Huang, E. J., Lipsitz, S., Pradarelli, J. C., Delisle, M., et al. (2020). Using smartphones to capture novel recovery metrics after cancer surgery. *JAMA Surgery, 155*(2), 123–129. https://doi.org/10.1001/jamasurg.2019.4702.

Seoane, E., & Hundt, M. (2018). Voice alternation and authorial presence: Variation across disciplinary areas in academic English. *Journal of English Linguistics, 46*(1), 3–22. https://doi.org/10.1177/0075424217740938.

Sword, H. (2012). *Stylish academic writing*. Cambridge, MA: Harvard University Press.

Urbach, D. R., Dimick, J. B., Haynes, A. B., & Gawande, A. A. (2019). Is WHO's surgical safety checklist being hyped? *BMJ, 366*, 4700. https://doi.org/10.1136/bmj.l4700.

Part III
The Community

Research is rarely a solo endeavor. The writing we use to disseminate our research, therefore, demands collaboration. Collaborative writing involves more than just writing: we describe how activities from brainstorming to editing make up the iterative process of writing as a group. Creating and sustaining teams that can write together isn't always easy, and in this section we offer some practical approaches to ensuring that collaborations support, rather than hinder, productivity. We address the delicate issue of interacting with our research peers, outlining strategies for that trickiest of conversations: the dreaded "response to reviews." We consider how research writers can band together, supporting each other through constructive feedback and targeted coaching. And we imagine how we might nurture writing communities that inspire, motivate, and raise everyone's game. We're stronger together.

Chapter 24
Collaborative Writing: Strategies and Activities

Scientific writing is rarely a solo act. It's not that the researcher doesn't sit the same lonely vigil as the novelist, hunched over her laptop at the kitchen table in a winter dawn, hoping for inspiration. Sure she does. But, unlike the novelist, the research writer is rarely the sole architect of the text she's creating. She is *sitting* alone at that table, but she is not *writing* alone. She writes on behalf of a team of collaborators, although she might wonder with the faintest tinge of resentment whether they are still in their warm beds as she sits in the pale morning light. Her sense of isolation is temporary, though. It will dissipate at the precise moment when five email messages ping into her inbox, each one offering its unique feedback and edits on her circulated draft.

Writing collaboratively can be the best of times and the worst of times. At best, it is richly rewarding. Collaborators brainstorm the vision of the piece together; they enhance the story by thoughtfully questioning one another's ideas; they craft the text iteratively, weaving a subtle tapestry of argument. At worst, it is deeply frustrating. Collaborators exchange ideas that don't cohere; they compete to pull the story in pet directions that both complicate and dilute it; they manufacture a stitched-together, Frankenstein of a text. Leading a collaborative writing effort, therefore, is a tricky business. And while many resources exist to help structure and support collaborative research (e.g., Bennett et al. 2010; Berndt 2011), most pay little attention to the activity of collaborative writing, beyond issues of authorship candidacy.

This chapter and the next aim to help you cultivate productive, satisfying writing relationships within your research team. In this chapter, we make explicit the strategies and activities involved when a group of researchers writes together, so that your research team can identify them and discuss how they will unfold in a particular project.

L. Lingard, C. Watling, *Story, Not Study: 30 Brief Lessons to Inspire Health Researchers as Writers*, Innovation and Change in Professional Education 19, https://doi.org/10.1007/978-3-030-71363-8_24

24.1   Strategies for Collaborative Writing

Collaborative writing is "an iterative and social process that involves a team focused on a common objective that negotiates, coordinates, and communicates during the creation of a common document" (Lowry et al. 2004, p 73). Collaborative writing can follow many different strategies (Ede and Lunsford 1990), but five are most common (Lowry et al. 2004). These are one-for-all writing, each-in-sequence writing, all-in-parallel writing, all-in-reaction writing, and multi-mode writing. Each offers a different approach to coordinating the work of writing in a group, and each is suited to different collaborative contexts.

One-for-all writing occurs when one person writes on behalf of the team. This strategy is appropriate when the writing task is simple and the stakes are low. For instance, many collaborative teams have a single author write an analytical memo describing the group's discussion at a research meeting. One-for-all writing offers stylistic consistency and efficiency, but can limit consensus building or revision unless these are explicitly built into document cycles. Therefore, it is best used by groups with a shared understanding of the writing task. Alternately, it can serve as an efficient, low-stakes way of producing a first rough draft that the team understands will undergo multiple iterations using a range of other writing strategies. Writing a first draft is, of course, never 'simple', but when the agreed goal is 'to get something on the page for us to work on together', one-for-all writing can work well.

Each-in-sequence writing occurs when one person starts the writing, completes their task and passes it on to the next person to complete theirs. This strategy is useful for groups working asynchronously who cannot meet often, and document-sharing platforms play a central role in its successful realization. Many teams will use it in the early stages of drafting a grant application, for instance, because it allows for straightforward coordination of distributed work. The sequence may be purposeful: for example, the lead author will draft the introduction of a manuscript, then the research assistant will draft the methods, then a third team member will draft the results, at which point the piece will return to the lead author to draft the discussion. In practice, however, the sequence is often more random: writers get to their sections when they can. Each-in-sequence writing introduces a number of challenges, including minimal social interaction, one-person bottlenecks, lack of coherence because differing ideas are not reconciled or writers invalidate one another's work, and haphazard version control. Together, these can result in poor overall coherence of the document. Teams can address these challenges by early meetings to clearly articulate the writing tasks and discuss areas of potential overlap or conflict. Also critical is agreement on the paper's main story and how it will thread through all sections, as well as a shared approach to writing style basics such as first or third person narration, and active or passive voice construction. Coherence is also improved by assigning a lead writer who oversees the sequence and takes responsibility for integration. However, this writer must have the authority to successfully fulfill this role (see next chapter).

All-in-parallel writing involves dividing the writing work into discrete units and writers working simultaneously rather than in sequence. This strategy works well in situations where the writing task is easily divided and individual sections are not mutually dependent. Because it tends to offer more process efficiency and writer autonomy than each-in-sequence writing, all-in-parallel writing can produce rapid, high volume output. The strategy is most effective when divisions of labor are not arbitrary but planned according to each writer's core expertise. For instance, the methodologist on a research team might write the first draft of the methods section, while a team member versed in the substantive domain of the work writes the literature review. The main challenge of all-in-parallel writing is that writers are blind to each other's work while writing, which can produce redundant or contradictory material. To mitigate this, parallel writing requires careful pre-planning, including an outline of how the parts relate to one another, a shared vision of the audience and purpose of the document, and a process to reconcile stylistic differences.

All-in-reaction writing involves researchers creating a document together in real time, adjusting to each other's changes and additions without explicit preplanning and coordination. Imagine, for example, that you write the first draft of a paper's Problem/Gap/Hook and send it to your co-authors simultaneously for review and response. They may make edits simultaneously, their edits may contradict or concur with you or with one another, and they may be carefully considered or spontaneous and impulsive. An advantage of the all-in-reaction collaborative writing strategy is that it can support consensus through fluid and creative expression of all team members. It can also provoke debates and enable new, unexpected meanings to emerge. Its main disadvantages include limited coordination, the potential for chaotic development of the piece, and difficulties with version control due to simultaneity of writing. And, for more novice or less powerful writers on the team, it can produce a turbulent, threatening experience. Therefore, all-in-reaction writing works best in small, non-hierarchical groups where all members feel safe to express their opinions. When these conditions are met, it can be a powerful strategy for interdisciplinary groups to create new meanings beyond the borders of conventional disciplinary thinking.

Multi-mode writing refers to when research teams use a combination of these strategies over the course of a writing project. For instance, a graduate student may produce the first draft of their research manuscript (one-for-all), which is then reviewed sequentially by team members, either as their calendars allow (each-in-random-sequence) or in a preplanned order (each-in-purposeful-sequence). Revisions are then produced by the graduate student (one-for-all), and each team member reviews closely one section of the revision according to their expertise (all-in-parallel). The abstract may be written (often mere hours before the conference submission deadline) on Google Docs or by flurry of emails, with all team members simultaneously helping to whittle the word count and prioritize the key messages (all-in-reaction). Ensuring that all writers are capable users of the technologies supporting the collaborative process is critical.

- What collaborative writing strategies does our team employ?
- Are our strategies purposeful, selected according to the nature of the team and the needs of the project, or are they accidental?
- Do we explicitly discuss how we will coordinate the work, or do we tacitly enact the same strategy each time?
- Are we using each strategy in ways that maximize its affordances and minimize its challenges?
- Are we using technology appropriately to support our collaborative activities?

Fig. 24.1 Questions for talking about collaborative writing strategies

These five strategies offer a framework for thinking critically about your own collaborative writing practices. Ask yourself questions such as those in Fig. 24.1.

Being purposeful and explicit about your collaborative writing strategy can help your team to maximize its unique affordances and minimize its challenges.

24.2 Activities of Collaborative Writing

Collaborative writing involves more than just *writing*. Writing researchers have identified seven core activities: brainstorming, conceptualizing, outlining, drafting, reviewing, revising, and editing. (Lowry et al. 2004).

In brainstorming, the writing group creates a list of potential ideas for the paper. Through conversation and text, they consider how to best represent the findings, what they might say about those findings in relation to the research question, what storylines would make for a compelling discussion, and what conversations the piece might join in the literature. Brainstorming may start while data collection and analysis are still underway, particularly in qualitative research using theoretical sampling methods.

The activity of conceptualizing involves coalescing and prioritizing brainstorming ideas to articulate the central story of the paper. Some ideas will be set aside as insufficiently mature or irrelevant to the study's main purpose; others will be pursued in ongoing analyses and reading of related theoretical and empirical literatures. When a study will yield more than one story, the process of conceptualizing must also consider the order and audiences of multiple manuscripts: which story should be told first? To whom?

Once the story is conceptualized, outlining is the process of detailing how it will unfold throughout the sections of the research manuscript genre. What needs to go in the introduction and what would be an unnecessary detour? What degree of detail should the methods include? Which results will be included and in what order? How will the discussion develop the ideas from the introduction? Outlining is an activity that can lend itself more readily to solo than to collaborative work. However, even if one writer takes the lead on outlining, the process should be visible to other members of the group. Talking through the outline in rough as a team, and then reviewing the outline created by the lead author, is one way to maximize both efficiency and input at this stage of the writing process.

In drafting, the outlined sections are flushed out into full sentences, paragraphs, and arguments. Create a realistic schedule for this activity; an outline can seem like it lays the whole paper out, but the devil is in the details. Will the literature review be organized chronologically or by points of view in the current scholarly conversation? How much theoretical framing should appear in the Introduction? How elaborate should the Methods be, and what is the appropriate balance of description and justification? How will main results be illustrated, and which data should appear in tables, figures or quoted excerpts? How will the storyline develop in the discussion, beyond summary of results and limitations? In fact, when you acknowledge the complexity of the writing that goes into even a rough first draft, it probably makes more sense to draft sections in blocks. Consider pairing Methods and Results, and Introduction and Discussion, for instance, as these represent, respectively, the study and the story.

Reviewing, revising, and editing usually occur in cycles. In reviewing, all members read draft material and provide feedback orally, by email, or in the text itself as track changes or comment boxes. Ideally, reviewing is a directed activity, in which members of the group are asked to focus on particular issues at specific points in the writing process. Revising involves the consideration, prioritization and integration of feedback from group members into the draft. Cycles of reviewing and revising will take place until the text is substantively complete, logically coherent, and rhetorically effective. Editing involves micro-level revisions for style, grammar, and flow, which may take place either as individual sections mature or when the entire document is judged complete. Editing at this level may be an activity best undertaken by one writer on the team, in order that the paper does not read as though it was written by several individuals.

These collaborative writing activities are dynamic and iterative. Sometimes the storyline needs revisiting after a particularly substantive round of reviewing. Reviewing may shift into revising. Or editing may take place on some completed sections while other sections are still being reviewed. Because of this, successful collaboration requires cultivating a shared understanding of which activity is being undertaken at any given time. Are you finished brainstorming, you've agreed on a conceptualization, and you're now ready to outline the paper? If one writer thinks so, but another is still in brainstorming mode, this can impede progress. Are some writers providing review feedback at the level of micro-editing, while others are grappling with the conceptualization of the story as it is emerging in the draft? Is reviewing of a one-for-all draft turning into all-in-reaction revising? Having a language to talk about the different activities involved in collaborative writing can help to identify and resolve such disparate orientations to the work. And keep in mind that these activities are not 'neutral'; they occur in the context of interpersonal dynamics on a research team. Collaborators mark, claim, defend, and redraw intellectual territory as they work through the various activities associated with the writing (Larsen-Ledet and Korsgaard 2019). Being attentive to enactment of territoriality throughout the writing process can help you focus on, rather than deflect, points of tension. Because within these may reside the team's best opportunities to produce incisive, boundary-pushing thinking.

Depending on the writing project, these seven activities will receive variable emphasis and attention. Some results clearly dictate the storyline, making brainstorming less necessary. Some conceptualizations are sufficiently detailed that outlining can be more perfunctory. Some writers edit as they go, making the editing process less extensive at the end. The value of identifying these activities is to reflect on your own processes: does your writing team tend to skip some of these steps, such as outlining, and to what effect? Do some members of your writing team engage in some activities, such as reviewing, but not in others? Not every writer on a team will engage centrally in every activity. But some degree of participation in all of these writing activities yields more satisfying and efficient collaboration. For instance, team members not involved in the brainstorming and conceptualizing activities may inappropriately reintroduce through their reviewing and revising of drafts a storyline that the team had agreed to reserve for another paper. When such tensions in the writing emerge purposefully among collaborators engaged in all activities, they represent important moments for reviewing earlier decisions and perhaps reconceptualizing the piece. However, when they emerge incidentally because some collaborators are unaware of earlier activities, they can be a source of frustration and inefficiency.

24.3   Conclusion

For your research collaboration to culminate in successful collaborative writing, you need to be able to break "writing" into its constituent activities and agree on strategies to coordinate them. This chapter offers a vocabulary to support you in this work.

See One, Do One, Teach One
1. Using Fig. 24.1 as a guide, talk with your team about the strategies you currently use to support your collaborative writing. Note which strategies you have tended to overlook, and create a plan to incorporate them into your writing process.
2. The next time your group meets (in person or virtually) to work on writing, explicitly name the activity you wish to engage in. For example:

   (a) "Today we're outlining the results. How will we organize and illustrate our findings?"
   (b) "I will be drafting this section and then sending it around for your feedback about how well I've realized our concept of the story – hold any text revisions for a later draft, please."

(continued)

3. When you run into tensions in the collaborative writing process, consult these lists of strategies and activities to help you diagnose the source of the tension and explicitly address it.

References

Bennett, L.M., Gadlin, H., & Levine-Finley, S. (2010). *Team science and collaboration: A field guide*. National Institutes of Health. https://www.cancer.gov/about-nci/organization/crs/research-initiatives/team-science-field-guide/collaboration-team-science-guide.pdf. Accessed 19 Sept 2020.

Berndt, A. E. (2011). Developing collaborative research agreements. *Journal of Emergency Nursing, 37*(5), 497–498. https://doi.org/10.1016/j.jen.2011.04.010.

Ede, L., & Lunsford, A. (1990). *Singular texts/plural authors: Perspectives on collaborative writing*. Carbondale: Southern Illinois University Press.

Larsen-Ledet, I., & Korsgaard, H. (2019). Territorial functioning in collaborative writing: Fragmented exchanges and common outcomes. *Computer Supported Cooperative Work (CSCW), 28*, 391–433. https://doi.org/10.1007/s10606-019-09359-8.

Lowry, P. B., Curtis, A., & Lowry, M. R. (2004). Building a taxonomy and nomenclature of collaborative writing to improve interdisciplinary research and practice. *The Journal of Business Communication, 41*(1), 66–99. https://doi.org/10.1177/0021943603259363.

Chapter 25
Collaborative Writing:
Roles, Authorship & Ethics

Perhaps the only thing sadder than failed love is a betrayed scientific collaboration.

–Dr. Doc

You might not expect the scientific world to have its own version of popular advice columnist *Dear Abby*, but it does (Gadlin and Bennett 2012, p. 495). And among the *Dear Dr. Doc* letters, a number deal with problems of collaboration and authorship on research teams. We have led many research teams over the course of our careers and we're happy to report that conflict has been rare. But when it does arise, it usually centers on one of three situations: team members' roles during the writing, their candidacy for authorship, and their placement in the author order. We have made a habit of talking about authorship early and often during research collaborations and, still, it can be a delicate dance. In this second chapter on Collaborative Writing, we provide strategies and shared vocabulary for productively addressing roles, authorship and ethics when you are writing in a group.

25.1 Roles in Collaborative Writing

Some of the most critical aspects of collaborative writing do not involve writing at all. Paramount among these are forming the writing group and articulating writers' roles.

Who is in the writing group? Research teams are getting larger and more complex, raising difficult questions about the relationship between the research team and the writing team. Sometimes the writing team is synonymous with the research team that wrote the grant, or collected and analyzed the data. Other times it is not. Subgroups may form to write different manuscripts, with research team members joining one or more subgroups based on availability and interest. Some individuals who had a key role in study procedures, such as research assistants, graduate students, or site leads, may have little or no role in the writing; in fact, they

L. Lingard, C. Watling, *Story, Not Study: 30 Brief Lessons to Inspire Health Researchers as Writers*, Innovation and Change in Professional Education 19, https://doi.org/10.1007/978-3-030-71363-8_25

> Carolyn was frustrated. She was the lead author on a conceptual paper being written by a collaboration among five mid-career scholars. The group was highly engaged, and Carolyn was struggling with the persistently conflicting feedback among the team related to fundamental issues like what would be the key storyline of the piece. After three rounds of drafting, review and revision, the paper still had not coalesced. Recognizing her frustration during the latest team Skype meeting to discuss the draft, another team member contacted her personally and offered this comment: "You are the lead author. You decide, and the team will honor that decision." This advice seemed to empower Carolyn. In the email accompanying the next draft, Carolyn wrote: "I have heard and considered all your feedback, and I'm grateful for your engagement. Here's what I've decided. ..." The next draft was substantially more coherent, and the team was supportive of her decisions.

Fig. 25.1 Leading the writing

may no longer be with the team at this point in the project. In other cases, one research team member may author a paper alone, such as when a PhD student writes a critical reflection on their emerging research identity in a project, or a principal investigator writes an invited commentary that draws on aspects of the research. The bottom line is that we cannot assume the membership of the writing group for a manuscript – we must explicitly discuss it.

There is no perfect configuration for a collaborative writing group. However, as the group grows in size and distribution (both geographical and disciplinary), the writing grows in complexity and difficulty. And, as many of us have experienced, often a small core of the larger writing group participates meaningfully in the seven activities described in the previous chapter, while other members participate only in reviewing drafts, with variable degrees of engagement. This raises the critical question of roles. What are the essential roles in a collaborative writing group? What degree of engagement is required to satisfy these roles?

First, every writing group needs a lead writer. Even in democratic writing collaborations where brainstorming, conceptualizing and drafting are shared, leadership is required to move the project forward (Frassl et al. 2018). Joint leadership is possible, particularly if the (likely two) individuals in this joint relationship employ some variations of all-in-parallel and all-in-reaction writing strategies, as we discussed in the previous chapter. The lead writer does not necessarily have to be the best writer in the group; in fact, in scientific writing, the lead writer is often a senior graduate student supervised by other members of the research team. However, the lead writer has to feel authorized to fulfill difficult aspects of their role, such as encouraging others' timely engagement, navigating conflicting ideas, and managing document control. Consider the example in Fig. 25.1.

When the lead writer is a graduate student or junior faculty member, support from a more senior team member may help to ensure that they succeed in fulfilling such aspects of the lead role. And, as Carolyn's example illustrates, even more senior team members may need their team's explicit support to enact the difficult decisions required in the lead author role.

Idina's research was going well. Data collection and analysis were completed, and the results were turning out to be even more exciting than the team had hoped. At the last team meeting they agreed that, even though the timing was tight, they would submit an abstract for an international conference whose deadline was only a week away. Idina drafted an abstract based on their conversation and circulated it the next day. By the submission date, two of her four collaborators had not responded and the other two had responded divergently: one commented 'great work!' in the margin while the other annotated the draft with substantive track changes and comment boxes. Idina was at a loss: should she make the changes suggested by the one team member and send the abstract in with all of their names attached? Should she circulate the substantially revised abstract for all to review and agree on submission? Should she remove from the abstract authorship those who had not offered feedback, given that she did not know if they agreed with the content? In the end, Idina decided that all co-authors should have the opportunity to review the substantially revised abstract and, since the looming deadline would not allow that to happen, she did not submit the abstract. At the next team meeting, the group discussed the feasibility of quick review cycles given the multiple commitments of many team members, and developed an agreement about how to handle time-sensitive non-responses in the future.

Fig. 25.2 Reconciling diverse feedback

The lead writer is a clear role in scientific writing; somewhat less clear is what everyone else should be doing. Will other team members also be involved in drafting, and if so, what is expected of them? Do they have ownership of that section until the work is complete, or does the lead author take over at the revision stage? Which team members will be reviewing, in what order, and with what focus? When feedback is discrepant, what process will be used to decide which suggestions to take up and which to set aside? Are all writers making conceptual contributions, or are some also making technical contributions such as formatting references or updating the literature review? When some or all of these issues are unclear, real quandaries can arise, as in Fig. 25.2.

Everyday issues complicate co-authorship, even when all team members have the best of intentions. Academic colleagues take on additional administrative roles that limit their availability. Clinical collaborators are unavailable for research during weeks of clinical service commitments. Graduate students complete their degrees and move. Research associates juggle multiple, part-time contract positions. Team members become ill, prioritize other commitments, lose interest in the project, or disagree with its direction. All of these can undermine the collaborative writing process. To ensure that all writers contribute meaningfully, discussing the roles of non-lead writers is an important part of planning in collaborative writing. Some recommend writing a joint contract to refer to if role expectations are not met as the writing proceeds, particularly in new or very large writing groups.

25.2   Authorship and Ethics

Authorship is the "coin of the realm" in scientific communities (Babor et al. 2017). According to sociologists of science, it is how we attribute credit, assign responsibility, and structure peer recognition in a reputation economy (Larivière et al. 2016). Co-authorship is an expanding phenomenon: Brand et al. (2015) reported that the average number of authors on scientific papers rose from two in the 1930s to seven by 2000, with author maximums in MEDLINE-indexed papers ranging from 38 pre-1975 to hundreds or even thousands in recent years (Larivière et al. 2016). Co-authorship is a highly contextualized system: lack of consistency in author ordering practices from one discipline to the next presents a particular problem in this age of interdisciplinary research collaborations (McFarlane 2017). Co-authorship is also a troubled system. Recent concerns include: the "white bull effect" in which senior authors coercively assert first authorship over junior authors (Kwok 2005); the global phenomenon of "hyperprolific" authors who publish a paper every 5 days (Ioannidis et al. 2018); and the problem of "gift" ordering in which authorship is ceded by a junior to a senior author based on a sense of indebtedness (McFarlane 2017). Health professions education research is not immune from such problems: recent reports have described honorary authorship (Uijtdehaage et al. 2018) and author misconduct in response to publication pressure (Maggio et al. 2019b).

How can you ensure that authorship is accurately and fairly represented in your collaboratively written manuscripts? Different guidelines exist, published by journals and academic organizations. However, in health research domains, most guidelines reflect the criteria put forward by the International Committee of Medical Journal Editors (ICMJE) Recommendations (ICMJE 2018). These are reproduced verbatim in Fig. 25.3.

When you use these criteria to support authorship conversations on your research team, keep in mind three things. First, the criteria are joined by "AND" (capitalization in original), rather than "or"; collaborators must fulfill all of them to qualify for authorship. Second, the criteria are not a rubric for disqualifying collaborators from authorship as a project proceeds. Collaborators who meet the first criterion should

---

Substantial contributions to the conception or design of the work; or the acquisition, analysis, or interpretation of data for the work;

AND

Drafting the work or revising it critically for important intellectual content;

AND

Final approval of the version to be published;

AND

Agreement to be accountable for all aspects of the work in ensuring that questions related to the accuracy or integrity of any part of the work are appropriately investigated and resolved.

Fig. 25.3 Authorship criteria from ICMJE Recommendations, Dec 2018 update

have the opportunity to meet the other three, which is another reason why you should think about authorship early on, when the research team is first assembled. Engaging a large team in the drafting and revising process requires an appropriate schedule and strategy for coordinating their input. Third, co-authors are not only responsible for their own contributions; each author is responsible for the whole and must "be able to identify which co-authors are responsible for specific other parts of the work" and "have confidence in the integrity of the contributions of their co-authors" (Smith et al. 2019, p. 2). If the paper becomes famous, everyone shares the glory; if it becomes infamous, everyone shares the blame and potential legal liability.

Once you have decided which of your team members have participated in ways that qualify for authorship, the thorny question of author order arises. Author order is a way of further nuancing the assignment of credit for the work. First and last author are the positions associated with highest credit for the work because they signal the most substantive contributions, a convention confirmed by a recent analysis of the contributor statements in >87,000 articles from multiple scientific disciplines (Ioannidis et al. 2018). When authorship disputes arise, they are usually about who deserves first author credit. This can be a difficult judgement, particularly in truly collaborative teams. Say one collaborator leads the project conceptualization overall, but another leads a substantial phase of analysis and interpretation leading to this paper: which one should be first author? One helpful principle is creativity (Dance 2012). For instance, if the analysis and interpretation produced a creative, original idea not represented in the original project conceptualization, this would be a rationale for assigning first authorship to the individual who led the analysis. If the two cannot be teased apart, co-first authorship may be a solution if the discipline or journal recognizes this variant. In co-first authorship, the first and second authors receive equal credit for the work.

First authors are often more junior collaborators, such as doctoral students and early career scientists, who lead the research and writing, while last authors may be more senior team members who scaffold, supervise and support the lead author. Teams should carefully distinguish between senior authorship for a team member who has played an authentic supervisory role, and "honorary" authorship for a department chair or research lab head who has benevolently supported the work from a distance. The latter would not meet the ICMJE criteria. Either first or senior authors may serve as the "corresponding author", a role that involves leading communications between the writing group and the scholarly community, as represented by the journal or individuals who write to respond to the paper. Authorship order "in the middle" is handled variously: it may reflect decreasing degrees of contribution or it may be alphabetic. The logic of middle ordering is usually implicit rather than explicit to readers of the manuscript, but the collaborative team should discuss and agree on it.

Authorship order has long been under fire as a way of representing collaborative work (e.g., Garfield 1982; Smith 1997; Martinson et al. 2005). The system is viewed as subjective and vulnerable to abuse, with author order reflecting politics or seniority as often as it does actual contribution. Junior team members may be particularly disadvantaged because for them the reputational stakes are especially

Over coffee, Gavin, a junior scientist, and his two office mates discuss how their Center Director appears as senior author on many of the publications produced by their group. Gavin wonders if such 'honorary' authorship might be expected on his current paper, given that the Director provided a letter of support for the successful grant application, gave thoughtful feedback at his lunchtime rounds presentation of his in-progress analysis, and often stops by his office doorway to ask how things are going. Gavin brings the concern to his next meeting with a senior member of his research team. They decide to send an email to the Director to deflect that possible expectation. The email, sent by Gavin and cc'd to his senior team member, provides an update on the progress of the work, a thanks for the Director's ongoing support, and the following sentence: "We would like to include an Acknowledgement in the paper to express our gratitude for the Department's support of this educational research initiative. May I send you a draft of the Acknowledgement text for your approval?" Gavin and his team figured that, even if it does not entirely deflect the expectation of honorary authorship, this strategy would make an explicit conversation necessary rather than allowing a tacit assumption to persist.

Fig. 25.4 Managing authorship expectations

high (Kwok 2005). So may team members whose contributions fit uneasily into the language of authorship guidelines, such as technicians who conduct lab procedures or librarians who set up search strategies for reviews (Strange 2008). Additionally, if one team member controls access to study data, others may find themselves "data hostages" to that individual's authorship demands (Maggio et al. 2019a).

Such situations have given rise to calls for new ways of authentically representing collaborative work, such as emphasizing contributorship over authorship and using acknowledgements for contributions that don't meet the authorship bar (Larivière et al. 2016). Regardless of what guideline or framework you apply, most important is the *conversation* about how that framework will apply to your team's activities. Researchers fear authorship discussions and therefore avoid them (Smith et al. 2019). How can you ensure that this doesn't happen on your team? One strategy is to include writing roles and authorship as standing items on your research team meeting agenda, so that you minimize the likelihood of unfortunate surprises at the time of manuscript conceptualization or submission. When the manuscript is being drafted, each author could write their own contribution statement according to the specific journal guidelines or, if those are lacking, according to general guidelines such as PLoS One's CRediT Taxonomy (PLoS One n.d.). Another strategy is to pro-actively deflect inappropriate expectations, as in the example in Fig. 25.4.

Perhaps the most powerful strategy for cultivating appropriate authorship expectations on a collaboration research team is role modelling by senior team members. When junior researchers see their doctoral supervisor or department chair saying, "I'm happy to offer my feedback on this paper but I don't qualify for or expect authorship as a result", this sends a clear message about the culture of authorship.

25.3   Conclusion

Writing roles and authorship should be discussed at the start of the research project and revisited as the analysis matures and the writing unfolds. Because these are high-stakes issues in collaborative health research, sensitive conversations may be necessary. Trying to avoid these uncomfortable interactions only defers them to critical moments, which increases the strain on the team and can irretrievably damage both the current collaboration and future research relationships. Instead, aim to develop a shared vocabulary and ongoing process for discussing these critical topics in your collaborative writing team.

See One, Do One, Teach One
1. Create a standing item on your team meeting agenda for Authorship.
2. Using the Authorship criteria from ICMJE Recommendations as a guide, have each team member draft a contributor statement for themselves. Discuss these together.
3. If your team is interdisciplinary, discuss the meaning of authorship order in your disciplines and strategize for how authorship order will be handled on your paper(s) to reflect these differing values.
4. Draft a plan for handling quick review cycles for upcoming conference abstract submissions.

References

Babor, T., Morisano, D., & Noel, J. (2017). Coin of the realm: Practical procedures for determining authorship. In T. F. Babor, K. Stenius, R. Pates, M. Miovský, J. O'Reilly, & P. Candon (Eds.), *Publishing addiction science: A guide for the perplexed* (pp. 207–227). London: Ubiquity Press.

Brand, A., Allen, L., Altman, M., Hlava, M., & Scott, J. (2015). Beyond authorship: Attribution, contribution, collaboration, and credit. *Learned Publishing, 28*(2), 151–155. https://doi.org/10.1087/20150211.

Dance, A. (2012). Authorship: Who's on first? *Nature, 489*, 591–593. https://doi.org/10.1038/nj7417-591a.

Frassl, M. A., Hamilton, D. P., Denfeld, B. A., de Eyto, E., Hampton, S. E., Keller, P. S., et al. (2018). Ten simple rules for collaboratively writing a multi-authored paper. *PLoS Computational Biology, 14*(11), e1006508. https://doi.org/10.1371/journal.pcbi.1006508.

Gadlin, H., & Bennett, L. M. (2012). Dear doc: Advice for collaborators. *Translational Behavioral Medicine, 2*(4), 495–503. https://doi.org/10.1007/s13142-012-0156-1.

Garfield, E. (1982, July 26). More on the ethics of scientific publication: Abuses of authorship attribution and citation amnesia undermine the reward system of science. *Essays of an information scientist* (Vol. 5). http://www.garfield.library.upenn.edu/essays/v5p621y1981-82.pdf. Accessed 16 Sept 2020.

International Committee of Medical Journal Editors. (2018). *Recommendations for the conduct, reporting, editing, and publication of scholarly work in medical journals.* http://www.icmje.org/icmje-recommendations.pdf. Accessed 14 Nov 2019.

Ioannidis, J. P. A., Klavans, R., & Boyack, K. W. (2018). Thousands of scientists publish a paper every five days. *Nature, 561*, 167–169. https://doi.org/10.1038/d41586-018-06185-8.

Kwok, L. S. (2005). The white bull effect: Abusive coauthorship and publication parasitism. *Journal of Medical Ethics, 31*, 554–556. https://doi.org/10.1136/jme.2004.010553.

Larivière, V., Desrochers, N., Macaluso, B., Mongeon, P., Paul-Hus, A., & Sugimoto, C. R. (2016). Contributorship and division of labor in knowledge production. *Social Studies of Science, 46*(3), 417–435. https://doi.org/10.1177/0306312716650046.

Maggio, L. A., Artino, A. R., Jr., Watling, C. J., Driessen, E. W., & O'Brien, B. C. (2019a). Exploring researchers' perspectives on authorship decision making. *Medical Education, 53*, 1253–1262. https://doi.org/10.1111/medu.13950.

Maggio, L., Dong, T., Driessen, E., & Artino, A., Jr. (2019b). Factors associated with scientific misconduct and questionable research practices in health professions education. *Perspectives on Medical Education, 8*, 74–82. https://doi.org/10.1007/s40037-019-0501-x.

Martinson, B. C., Anderson, M. S., & de Vries, R. (2005). Scientists behaving badly. *Nature, 435*, 737–738. https://doi.org/10.1038/435737a.

McFarlane, B. (2017). The ethics of multiple authorship: Power, performativity and the gift economy. *Studies in Higher Education, 42*(7), 1194–1210. https://doi.org/10.1080/03075079.2015.1085009.

PLoS One. (n.d.). *Authorship*. https://journals.plos.org/plosone/s/authorship. Accessed 5 Feb 2020.

Smith, R. (1997). Authorship: Time for a paradigm shift? *BMJ, 314*, 992. https://doi.org/10.1136/bmj.314.7086.992.

Smith, E., Williams-Jones, B., Master, Z., Larivière, V., Sugimoto, C. R., Paul-Hus, A., et al. (2019). Researchers' perceptions of ethical authorship distribution in collaborative research teams. *Science and Engineering Ethics, 26*(4), 1995–2022. https://doi.org/10.1007/s11948-019-00113-3.

Strange, K. (2008). Authorship: Why not just toss a coin? *American Journal of Physiology-Cell Physiology, 295*(3), C567–C575. https://doi.org/10.1152/ajpcell.00208.2008.

Uijtdehaage, S., Mavis, B., & Durning, S. J. (2018). Whose paper is it anyway? Authorship criteria according to *established* scholars in health professions education. *Academic Medicine, 93*(8), 1171–1175. https://doi.org/10.1097/ACM.0000000000002144.

Chapter 26
Giving Feedback on Others' Writing

Recently, a medical educator colleague of ours did a remarkable thing. In an effort to illuminate coaching practices for fellow medical teachers, he called upon his experience as a musician, staging a live cello master class and featuring himself as the learner. He's already a fine musician, but his coach wanted him to bring some emotional depth to his playing – a quality in the performances of great musicians that we might be inclined to think of as intangible, even unteachable. She didn't simply tell him to play with more emotion, however. Instead, she talked about the pressure on the bow, the arc of the bow stroke, the movement of his body, the position of the bow on the strings, and the way he handled tempo and dynamics. She deconstructed "emotion" into its component technical parts, and our colleague's playing transformed in front of our eyes.

While this master class was about music, it mirrored the challenge and the joy of giving others feedback on their writing. Most of us not only write, but also read, edit, critique, and support the writing of students or colleagues. Handled poorly, feedback on writing can be confusing, unhelpful, and even discouraging. But handled well, feedback on writing – like feedback on cello playing – has the power to transform. In this chapter, we offer guidance for harnessing this power.

26.1 Focus Your Efforts

Ideally, feedback should feel like a conversation between reader and writer. To achieve this, it helps to establish what the conversation is going to be about. Writers should make focused requests of their readers, such as "I'd like to know if my Problem/Gap/Hook is clear in the opening paragraph" or "I'm wondering if my paragraph transitions are working" or "I'm concerned the discussion just repeats the results but I'm not sure how to fix it". When writers don't make specific requests, readers should ask for direction: "What would you like me to focus on? Logic of the

L. Lingard, C. Watling, *Story, Not Study: 30 Brief Lessons to Inspire Health Researchers as Writers*, Innovation and Change in Professional Education 19, https://doi.org/10.1007/978-3-030-71363-8_26

argument? Sentence and paragraph construction? Success with achieving a particular tone?" Writers and readers who are unsure about where to focus their feedback conversations might consider the three editing targets we described in Chap. 19: attending first to story, then to structure, and finally to style offers one useful strategy for organizing feedback. Whatever the strategy, agreeing on a focus is critical. When a writer needs feedback about whether or not their storyline is sufficiently compelling, the last thing they'll want is a grammar lesson. Feedback that doesn't align with a writer's needs is unlikely to land, even if accurate.

Even with focused requests for feedback, readers will almost certainly notice other aspects of the writing that need strengthening. What if that grammar lesson, unwelcome as it may be, is badly needed? Remember that writers can only absorb so much feedback at once. Maintain your focus on a few areas and just note other issues to be addressed in future. For instance, if you see that a writer struggles to use commas appropriately, flag one or two in the draft and add a comment box that says you will address this grammar issue later. Or, if the tone of the writing is too casual for a research manuscript, mention that this is something to discuss a few drafts further along. Put a pin in the issue, without overwhelming the writer with too much feedback at once.

26.2 Be Specific

Agreeing on a feedback focus is necessary but not sufficient for success. In addition, your actual comments on the writing need to be specific in order to be actionable. This can be quite tricky. Many readers possess good instincts for when something is wrong with the writing and know how to fix it themselves. But many also lack the vocabulary and knowledge to *name* the problem and *explain* the fix. Lacking this, readers default to offering generic comments ("awkward", "unclear", and "vague" are favorites) or fixing the problem without commenting at all. Neither approach helps the writer to diagnose and solve their recurring writing weaknesses.

What is the reader who is not a writing expert to do? First, use the chapters in this book to help you to diagnose and name the problems you can. For instance, instead of scribbling "confusing" beside a paragraph, remind the writer about paragraph structure: "A paragraph needs an opening topic sentence to orient the reader to its main idea, and that idea should develop as the paragraph unfolds. I think either your topic sentence is missing, or it's the wrong topic sentence for this paragraph, or the paragraph just includes too many ideas." Second, when your instinct tells you something isn't working but you're not sure why, just say so. For instance, many writers create long, meandering sentences that lose the reader, but you might not know exactly what's gone grammatically wrong. In such cases, share your reading experience: "This very long sentence lost me about here. You could try breaking it into 2 or 3 sentences or using stronger punctuation to help the reader follow the relationships between these ideas."

26.3   Engage the Writer

Comments like these remind us that giving feedback on someone's work and editing someone's work are two different tasks. When offering feedback, try to resist the urge to simply rewrite. Think about making comments for consideration, rather than making changes that the writer can simply accept. Rampant use of the "track changes" function in Word may reduce the likelihood of the writer really engaging with the feedback. Sometimes all a writer is looking for is some careful copy editing. But if they've asked for feedback, provide it in a way that they can really engage with the process. If a writer's paragraph is unconvincing, for example, try something like: "This key paragraph isn't as compelling as it could be. The problem may be that you have used a lot of 'to be' verbs. Try replacing a few of them with stronger, action-oriented verbs to better command the reader's attention." There's a much greater chance the writer will be able to use your feedback in other situations if you highlight concerns, offer possible diagnoses, articulate an option or two for improvement, and provide a rationale for your suggestions.

Although mere rewriting can be dispiriting, a demonstration of how your feedback can be put to work can be powerful. Therefore, aim for a balance of telling and showing in your feedback. If you use a rewrite to show how a passage may be strengthened, couple your edits with an explanatory note. For example, because parallel structure is an effective device for strengthening the impact of writing, you might wordsmith a paragraph to inject a dose of parallelism. Nothing wrong with that – but the rewrite is much more effective as feedback if accompanied by a comment that explains, "I've tried to create a parallel structure here by matching the grammatical construction of the first three sentences. I think this change makes the ideas more persuasive."

26.4   Tread Carefully

Remember that writing – even academic writing – can be deeply personal. Feedback on writing, therefore, is a delicate business; a critique of writing as product can easily be misinterpreted as a critique of writer as person. When feedback threatens self-esteem or stirs strong emotions, it becomes very challenging for individuals to process and integrate, even if it is accurate and potentially useful (Kluger and DeNisi 1996; Sargeant et al. 2008). Advice about feedback typically encourages us to focus on the task rather than on the individual in order to defuse threats to self-esteem and mitigate negative emotion (Lefroy et al. 2015). But because the task of writing is not emotionally neutral, this may be easier said than done. Acknowledging this challenge honestly may be helpful. Focusing on the experience of the reader also helps; for example, instead of saying "Your use of jargon is confusing", consider instead "I'm worried that some readers may not understand these terms – perhaps a definition would help here."

A little praise doesn't hurt either. Look for strengths and successes to point out to the writer, like "what a powerful verb!", "lovely turn of phrase here", "strong transitions between these paragraphs", or "nice job balancing a formal research tone with more conversational moments". Such feedback reinforces good practice and bolsters confidence, and we all need our writing confidence bolstered! When you are working closely with a writer and seeing multiple drafts, you have the opportunity to comment specifically on improvements from past drafts. This signals to the writer that her efforts to change were worth it, that she is gaining expertise, and that pleasing you is not a random event. We say the last only partly tongue-in-cheek, because we know that writers may perceive contradictions in multiple rounds of feedback on their writing. Sometimes, as the drafts evolve, we readers change our minds. This is okay; in fact it can be very instructive for writers *if* the reasoning is explicit. After all, successful writing is a craft, not a recipe. In this spirit, we have found ourselves writing comments that admit, "I know I suggested to try this new organization, but I don't think it's working. The logic seems to fall apart. I propose we go back to the earlier structure but put more emphasis on explicit signposting to make it easier for readers to follow."

This last example highlights the value of humility when offering feedback. Many of us wonder whether or not we will be seen as credible when we provide feedback on others' writing, particularly when we are dealing with experienced colleagues. Molloy and Bearman (2019) describe a quality they call "intellectual candour", which involves the expression of doubt and uncertainty to support teaching and learning around complex problems. Intellectual candor is an expression of vulnerability from the teacher that may level the playing field, inviting reciprocal vulnerability from the learner (Molloy and Bearman 2019). Applied to writing feedback, this notion suggests that when we share the struggles and dilemmas that plague our own writing, the quality of our feedback conversations will be enhanced. We position ourselves alongside our feedback recipients in grappling with the shared problem of writing effectively, and we model the guiding principle that we are all trying to become better writers.

26.5   Conclusion

Writing feedback is a powerful tool. Use it consciously, and with care. At the end of our colleague's cello master class, one of the audience members asked the teacher about her philosophy when giving feedback to musicians. She thought for a moment, then said "You must be sure that you don't kill the joy." Writing, like playing music, can be technical and frustrating. But it can also be joyous, and supporting writers to find that joy may be the key to sustaining their engagement in the challenging craft of writing.

See One, Do One, Teach One

1. The next time you are asked to provide feedback on a draft, make a point of having a conversation first that establishes the ground rules for the feedback. What is it that the writer would like you to focus on? Is there anything they don't wish feedback on? How will you handle issues that require attention but that aren't within the scope of what was requested?
2. Try offering feedback on a draft with the "Track changes" function turned OFF. Use comment boxes instead, which may force you to suggest and instruct more than you rewrite.
3. Ask a trusted colleague for feedback on your feedback. Before you send your feedback back to the writer, ask your colleague these questions:

   (a) Have I been specific in naming problems?
   (b) Would the writer be able to act on this feedback?
   (c) Are there opportunities for me to provide examples of what I'm getting at that I have overlooked?
   (d) How's the balance of critique and praise?

References

Kluger, A. N., & DeNisi, A. (1996). The effects of feedback interventions on performance: A historical review, a meta-analysis, and a preliminary feedback intervention theory. *Psychological Bulletin, 119*(2), 254–284. https://doi.org/10.1037/0033-2909.119.2.254.

Lefroy, J., Watling, C., Teunissen, P. W., & Brand, P. (2015). Guidelines on feedback for clinical education: The dos, don'ts, and don't knows of feedback for clinical education. *Perspectives on Medical Education, 4*(6), 284–299. https://doi.org/10.1007/s40037-015-0231-7.

Molloy, E., & Bearman, M. (2019). Embracing the tension between vulnerability and credibility: 'Intellectual candour' in health professions education. *Medical Education, 53*(1), 32–41. https://doi.org/10.1111/medu.13649.

Sargeant, J., Mann, K., Sinclair, D., van der Vleuten, C., & Metsemakers, J. (2008). Understanding the influence of emotions and reflection upon multi-source feedback acceptance and use. *Advances in Health Science Education, 13*, 275–288. https://doi.org/10.1007/s10459-006-9039-x.

Chapter 27
Coaching Writing I:
Being Thoughtful About the Process

Every health researcher gives feedback on others' writing. Usually we do so as co-authors, supervisors, or pre-submission 'barometer' readers. Such feedback almost always makes writing better, and the previous chapter offered strategies to maximize its effectiveness. Sometimes, however, we're doing more than providing feedback on a draft. Sometimes we're coaching other researchers as writers.

"Coaching" is not a word that health researchers commonly use in relation to their writing, so you might need to stop and think about this for a minute. Do you have someone who reads most if not all of your writing, who knows your writing processes as well as your products, who has helped you evolve as a writer? Or perhaps you *are* that person for a peer, junior colleague or graduate student: is there someone whose 'voice' you have watched develop over many manuscripts? Someone whose writing style you recognize well enough to know when they're trying something new or struggling with a longstanding challenge?

Chances are that you will have said 'Yes!' (or 'Hmmm, maybe . . .') to one or all of these questions. Now ask yourself, is that coaching relationship purposeful or accidental? Accidental doesn't necessarily mean ineffective, but we believe that writing coaching is empowered when it is conscious, explicit and planned. Evidence suggests that writing coaching can improve health researchers' productivity and their satisfaction (Baldwin and Chandler 2002). We conceptualize writing coaching around three domains – process, relationship, and identity. This chapter focuses on process, the next on relationship and identity. Together, they offer tips to help you create positive coaching interactions.

© The Author(s), under exclusive license to Springer Nature Switzerland AG 2021
L. Lingard, C. Watling, *Story, Not Study: 30 Brief Lessons to Inspire Health
Researchers as Writers*, Innovation and Change in Professional Education 19,
https://doi.org/10.1007/978-3-030-71363-8_27

27.1   Five Process Tips for Sound Coaching

All writing coaching centers around a particular piece of writing. Coaching writing, however, is distinct from giving feedback on a piece of writing. In fact, our first two tips for writing coaching involve knowing when to set the writing aside:

Work on the Thinking

Writing is not the only product you're working on together. As historian David McCullough put it, "Writing is thinking ... that's why it's so hard" (Cole 2002). Particularly when you are giving multiple rounds of feedback on work-in-development, you are coaching the thinking as well as the writing. It is important to step back and be explicit about which is in the foreground at any point in time. Try telling the writer, "I think this is a snarl in the thinking/logic more than a problem with the writing. Let's play with that a bit more."

When you want to play with the thinking, it can also be helpful to:

Talk It Out

Speaking is a powerful adjuvant to writing. When you find yourselves at a conceptual crossroads (or, even worse, deep in a conceptual swamp), put the draft aside and chat about the story. Brainstorm, play with the ideas, summarize back to each other what you think you understand. It can be easier to relinquish past ideas and structures when you haven't committed them to the page. Audio record these sessions if it's helpful for the writer, but the goal is not phrasing you can cut and paste into a draft: it's coherence of ideas.

Coaching begins with the written product. But when you need to work on the thinking, a conversation can move things forward. Many of us are more confident conversationalists than we are writers: capitalize on that to minimize stress and focus attention on the ideas.

Unlike writing feedback, writing coaching extends beyond a single piece of writing. Coaches and writers engage in a longitudinal process that spans multiple manuscripts. Therefore, coaching has the ability – indeed, the responsibility – to also address writing process. We offer two tips, with supporting models from the literature, to help with this aspect of coaching.

Address Attitudes about Writing

Writing success happens in the head before it translates to the page. Good writers talk themselves into writing, whether they feel like it or not, whether they know what to write or not, whether they like or hate what they see appearing on the screen. Keeping on, even when the writing starts ugly (as so much writing does!), is the key. Writers have to *believe*. Therefore, coaches need to understand writers' beliefs about writing.

Gardiner and Kearns' ABCDE model is a useful approach to exploring beliefs about writing. Based on cognitive behavioral coaching, it aims to change writing practice by targeting the underlying beliefs of the writer. It is based on the premise

Table 27.1 Common writing beliefs and consequences

Beliefs	Consequences
It's too soon; I'm not ready to write yet.	I'll wait. Next week looks like a better time.
I need to get the paper clear in my head before I start.	I think I'll read a bit more.
I don't have enough time.	I'll email my co-authors & set up a meeting.
What I write won't be good anyway.	I'll clean my closet.

Table 27.2 Some common writer thoughts and their disputation

Readiness		Clarity		Quality	
Thoughts	Disputation	Thoughts	Disputation	Thoughts	Disputation
I'm not in the mood.	Your mood often shifts once you get started writing.	*It needs to be clear in my head first.*	Writing can help make things clearer.	*It won't be good enough.*	You've written good work before, you can again.
I don't have enough time.	A little time can yield a surprising amount.	*I just need to think for a bit longer.*	Think about what you've written after.	*It's got a lot of mistakes.*	All drafts have mistakes. Focus on 1 thing to improve.
It should come naturally.	All writers struggle; the 'natural' is a myth.	*I don't know how to start.*	Start where it's easiest: Methods maybe?	*If I share this, it will expose me as a fraud.*	It's called imposter syndrome. We all have it. You're not a fraud.

that, faced with the "Activating event" of a looming writing task, many researchers will be influenced by their underlying Beliefs, which in turn give rise to unhelpful Consequences that impede effective writing. Common beliefs and consequences are outlined in Table 27.1, adapted from Gardiner and Kearns (2012).

Beliefs about writing tend to cluster around three issues: readiness, clarity, and quality. The ABCDE model turns on the "Disputation" stage: helping the writer to recognize the inaccuracy of the thoughts they have based on these three beliefs. Disputing these thoughts by drawing on facts is the first step towards changing them. Table 27.2, adapted from Gardiner and Kearns (2012), illustrates how writers' common thoughts about readiness, clarity and quality can be disputed:

By disputing common thoughts about writing, coaches can help writers adopt new ways of thinking, which lead to an Effective new outlook and behavior. The goal is to shift beliefs so that writers get started writing and "stay started". Regular, daily writing in whatever time increments are possible is the key. By using the ABCDE model to reflect on what's going on in the writer's head that influences writing process, coaches can help writers to develop a sense of self-efficacy and keep their limiting beliefs at bay.

Time
- What is your writing routine? Daily, weekly, monthly? Do you have a routine?
- How much time do you spend writing during each session?
- At what time of day do you usually write? Why?
- Have you tried writing at a different time?

Space
- What is your physical writing spot like in terms of comfort, clutter, privacy, aesthetics?
- What are the main distractions in your physical conditions? How can you modify them?
- Have you tried writing in a different space? Outside instead of inside? In an easy chair rather than at a desk? Without windows? Without wifi?

Ritual
- What do you do when you first sit down to write? What do you do at each session's end?
- What do you do when you hit a roadblock?
- Are you engaged in the process of writing or the process of revising your writing? How do you distinguish these processes?
- What metaphors do you use when you think or talk about your writing? Are you 'juggling' multiple writing projects or 'focusing' on one until complete? Do you plan meticulously, like an architect, or more organically, like a gardener?

Fig. 27.1 Reflecting on time, space, & ritual

Talk About the Physical Conditions of the Writing

Good writing practice is the product of multiple conditions, many of which we never subject to critical scrutiny. Things like when and where we write can have powerful, and largely unnoticed, impacts on our process.

Figure 27.1 offers a series of questions, adapted from Helen Sword's (2017) treatment of the "behavioral habits" of "time, space and ritual".

We encourage coaches and writers to use these questions, and create their own, to spark conversations about the physical and behavioral aspects of their writing process.

Finally, each of these process tips relies on coaches and writers taking the time to:

Engage in Reflection

Every writer knows how to perseverate on their writing: they agonize, they flog, they worry, they spin. But it can be difficult to reflect, productively and authentically, on their writing. Coaching, with its ability to analyze, to question, to offer alternatives, can help writers learn to reflect productively.

Coaching should encourage reflection at all stages of the writing process. By asking writers questions – Why do you feel that way about writing? How have you come to organize your writing projects this way? Why do you think reviewers reacted as they did? Why do you think it's difficult for you to change this habit? –

coaches help writers to develop a critical stance on their own process. Coaches also engage in self-reflection: How effective was that strategy I suggested? Have I amplified this writer's voice or made it sound like my own? Why do I feel so strongly about this advice?

27.2   Conclusion

Many health researchers give and receive feedback on writing. When this activity extends over multiple manuscripts and we approach it with a sense of purpose, writing feedback can be elevated to writing coaching. Writing coaching has much to offer health researchers, and we hope that these process tips can support more researchers to engage in it.

> **See One, Do One, Teach One**
> 1. Using Table 27.1 as a resource, have a coaching conversation to identify strong beliefs about writing and their consequences.
> 2. Using Table 27.2 as a resource, have a conversation to dispute the beliefs about readiness, clarity and quality that might be holding the writer back.
> 3. Using Fig. 27.1 as a resource, do an analysis of your behavioral habits as a writer.

References

Baldwin, C., & Chandler, G. (2002). Improving faculty publication output: The role of a writing coach. *Journal of Professional Nursing, 18*(1), 8–15. https://doi.org/10.1053/jpnu.2002.30896.

Cole, B. (2002). A visit with historian David McCullough. *Humanities, 24*(3).

Gardiner, M., & Kearns, H. (2012). The ABCDE of writing: Coaching high-quality high-quantity writing. *International Coaching Psychology Review, 7*(2), 247–259.

Sword, H. (2017). *Air and light and time and space: How successful academics write.* Cambridge, MA: Harvard University Press.

Chapter 28
Coaching Writing II: Relationship and Identity

Coaching writing isn't just about the writing. It's about the people. Whether the writer is a health research student and the coach their supervisor, or the writer and the coach are research peers, coaching works best when attention is paid to the relationship and its impact on the researcher's identity as a writer. This chapter offers six tips to help you be thoughtful about both.

First, though, a note about the ideal writing coach. She isn't necessarily an expert in the writer's content domain, although she needs to have experience with the genres (e.g., IMRD manuscript) in which the writer is working. And she also isn't necessarily a 'better' writer than those she coaches. In fact, some of the best writers are unable to say how they do it: their expertise is tacit (McGrath et al. 2019) and therefore they do not make good coaches. Like a good athletic coach, the writing coach's prowess lies in her ability to break the performance down into its component parts, offer critical analysis and actionable advice, work on the mental game underlying the performance, and support personal growth.

28.1 Using Relationships to Support Writing Development

Coaching is a relationship. And, because writing – even research writing – can be deeply personal, writing coaching is a high-stakes, intimate relationship. The first three tips in this chapter are strategies to establish and maintain a strong relationship between writer and coach.

Get to Know Each Other as Writers

Share a piece of your own writing that you're proud of. Discuss a paper you found particularly effective. Talk about your writing aspirations – such as your goal to publish original research in the *BMJ* – and your struggles – such as those paragraphs that take a whole day to write only to be deleted the next morning. Such sharing

© The Author(s), under exclusive license to Springer Nature Switzerland AG 2021
L. Lingard, C. Watling, *Story, Not Study: 30 Brief Lessons to Inspire Health Researchers as Writers*, Innovation and Change in Professional Education 19,
https://doi.org/10.1007/978-3-030-71363-8_28

demystifies writing for novices. It also explicitly rejects the culture of secrecy and competitiveness around academic writing that can make it inhospitable to new-comers (Aitchison 2018).

Create a Safe Space

Coaches need to provide a safe place for writers to develop, to confront their insecurities, to challenge themselves to be better, to become confident enough to improvise within the rules and to find their own voices. Give writers permission to submit messy drafts when the focus is more on thinking. Manage expectations by acknowledging that there will be many rounds of drafting and feedback before a final product emerges. Agree on the focus for a particular round of writing review – story, structure, or style (see Chap. 19) – and overlook the other aspects for now. Share reviewers' comments and discuss how to interpret and respond to them.

To reap the benefits of coaching, a writer needs to be willing to be vulnerable. As Molloy and Bearman (2019) note with reference to transformative learning in healthcare domains, expressing vulnerability is always in tension with maintaining credibility. They suggest "intellectual candour" as a way of building trust in this context. To enact intellectual candor, the coach must surface their own "inner struggles as a means of inviting reciprocal vulnerability" (p. 32). For example, coaches may share uncertainties about a manuscript that they've had rejected more than once, or they may reflect on difficulties they've experienced developing a powerful writing voice.

Coaching relationships have a trajectory. At the beginning, getting to know each other and creating a safe space are critical to establishing a productive coaching relationship. But the middle needs attention too. Maintaining a thriving coaching relationship as the writing and the writer evolve is not automatic: many relationships falter (or even fester) if the participants don't expect and allow the dynamic to change. Therefore, it is also important to:

Clarify Roles and Revisit Them Regularly

The roles of coach and writer are not static: they may need to be refreshed with reference to the specific writing task, the writer's stage of development, and the trajectory of the relationship. Making roles explicit and then revisiting them as the context evolves will help the coaching relationship stay relevant.

"Coach" is not a singular role. It can range from "critical friend" reviewing the coherence of a paragraph, "collaborator" working jointly on getting the layout of the results just right, "teacher" offering instruction on how to achieve a more appropriate register, or "gatekeeper" judging whether the work is adequate for submission (Wellington 2010). It's important to be clear which role you're playing. For instance, in a recent coaching interaction with an early career researcher, they suggested that they were ready to submit the manuscript for peer review. Lorelei's response went something like this: "It doesn't feel ready yet to me. Part of my role is as gatekeeper: there's a bar this needs to get over before it's ready for formal peer review. If you send it too soon, you risk damaging your reputation as a researcher and a writer."

The graduate supervisor role deserves specific mention here. Graduate supervision should always involve some degree of writing coaching over the course of the student's scholarly development. For those who have multiple graduate students or junior colleagues for whom they provide writing coaching, you might consider producing an introductory document to guide expectations and provide a foundation for conversations about how the relationship will work (e.g., Vanstone 2017). Keep in mind, though, that you will need to tailor your roles and expectations to the unique situation of each writer.

Outside the graduate supervisor role with its clear start and end, the coaching role can be a bit murky. You might wonder: "Am I coaching this writer?"; "Am I *still* coaching this writer?"; "Am I coaching this writer *in this situation*?" For clarity, it's worth spelling out a few "don'ts" about the coaching role. First, don't coach unless you've been asked to. You may think a co-author would benefit from coaching, but their explicit request for feedback on a draft is not a tacit invitation to coach. Second, don't make the mistake of thinking "once a coach, always a coach". Coaching relationships evolve and end: if the individuals continue to interact as colleagues or co-authors, coaches must take care to not to continue to invoke the coach role. Similarly, when coaches and writers have concurrent relationships as co-authors or colleagues, they should be explicit about how the intimacy and confidentiality of the coaching relationship will be handled alongside these other relationships.

28.2 Writing Identity Into Being

For the academic scholar, writing is a fundamental aspect of identity formation. We "write [our] identity into being" (Aitchison 2018, p. 193), and it's no easy task. The literature is replete with evidence that writing is a site of struggle for novice academics (Wellington 2010). At first we (and others) don't like how we sound, and it's a long, arduous process to learn first how to sound 'right' and then how to sound 'like myself'. This is why any scholar looks back a bit cringingly on their earliest publications -- we are not the same writers we were back then. Writing ourselves into being never stops.

Health researchers may particularly struggle to develop their writing identity. The identity formation literature focuses on the challenges for doctoral and postdoctoral trainees, but we would argue that developing a writer identity may be even more difficult for health researchers. Many years of health professional training create a wide gap between past writing instruction (often high school English) and current writing needs. This gap is not only temporal but also rhetorical: the early instruction likely does not translate readily to the requirements of the IMRD manuscript for a health research journal. For this reason, coaches need to spend sufficient time addressing health researchers' attitudes about writing (see Chap. 27). Confidence as a healthcare provider does not translate automatically into confidence as a health researcher nor, in our experience, into confidence as a writer. On the contrary, the dissonance between the identities of high-achieving, effective, respected healthcare provider and struggling, novice writer can be profound. Therefore, coaching in these circumstances must:

Respect the Vulnerability of Identity Formation

This vulnerability is real; however, it may remain invisible and tacit unless coaches name it and invite it into the interaction.

Coaches can try to notice when writers seem particularly vulnerable: they might even get into the habit of asking, "How challenging does this feel for you?" Similarly, coach and writer might set an explicit expectation for the writer to flag when something is particularly difficult or threatening. Without such attention, coaches can feel they are being enthusiastic and responsive, while writers just feel naked and exposed. Because recent research on coaching highlights failure as a powerful catalyst for learning (Watling and LaDonna 2019), coaches might share their own failures as a strategy for acknowledging and supporting the writer's "reciprocal vulnerability" (Molloy and Bearman 2019, p. 32). In our own coaching relationships, we make a point of talking about our "shitty first drafts" (Lamott 1994, p 21), harsh feedback experiences, and desk-rejected manuscripts. Not just because misery loves company, but also because vulnerability is a prerequisite for growth. And we are *all* growing as writers. Any writer who thinks otherwise will never be as good as she could have been.

A developing writer's vulnerability is compounded by struggles with language. Many health researchers write in English as an Additional Language (EAL). When coaching these writers, pay attention to how language affects the writer's sense of identity. For instance, EAL writers may feel that they have a recognizable voice as a writer in their first language, but that this is lost when they write in English. Coaches might ask such writers to write a list of adjectives that describe their voice, and have a conversation about how that is being achieved in the first language and how it might be translated to English.

Helping health researchers to develop a sense of themselves *as writers* is our ultimate aspiration as writing coaches. This is perhaps the most sophisticated aspect of writing coaching:

Realize a Complex and Coherent Voice

Identity is almost always multi-faceted. Writing coaching, therefore, supports the writer to recognize how their multiple identities influence their work and to represent that in their prose.

For example, if we were to coach a health researcher who is a family physician, a clinical educator and classical musician with a passion for arts and humanities, our goal would be to see those identities woven together in their writing. We might ask them to talk about music as a way of getting to know the images and metaphors that they use to express that aspect of their identity. If they write in other genres, such as commentaries about art and medicine, we would ask if we could discuss them. Many novice writers believe they need to expunge these other identities from their research manuscripts, but the goal should not be homogeneous prose. Rather, it should be credible, compelling, coherent prose. And coherent, here, means both internally coherent logic and coherence with who the writer *is*. If we can succeed in helping writers develop such writing identity, they will, we believe, find their writing more enjoyable.

Finally, we offer this advice as a fundamental principle for coaching relationships:

Remember, It's Ultimately about the Writer

Coaches offer advice, expertise, and support, but what writers do with those offerings is up to them. Coaches can become quite invested in the work, coming to see it as a reflection of their identity. This is understandable, but important to acknowledge and navigate carefully.

Consider the earlier example: there is a fine line between taking on the gatekeeper aspect of the coach role and taking over ownership of the writing. It can be helpful to think about these moments in terms of your "threshold of principles and preferences" (Apramian et al. 2015, p. 71). For instance, having a coherent story in a research paper is a principle for us (as we hope this book makes clear), but having a compelling metaphor that captures the main idea is a preference for Lorelei. Another coach may not share that preference. When we find ourselves in the zone of fiddling with preferences, it's time to remind ourselves that it is not our writing. Similarly, if the paper starts to sound like the coach rather than the writer, then that is a sign that the threshold between principle and preference has been crossed. If you find yourself here as a coach (and trust us, you will, despite the best laid plans), step back and have a discussion with the writer about what has happened and why. Remember, central to a great coaching performance is drawing out another person's unique character and skill, not duplicating your own.

28.3 Conclusion

The best coaches – in sports, in music – are judged not by their own performance, but by the performances of those they coach. If we can coach writing well, by attending carefully to process, relationship, and identity, then we stand to make health researchers more productive and skilled, to give them confidence in their identity *as writers*, and to infuse their writing work with satisfaction and joy.

See One, Do One, Teach One
1. Ask each other, "What kind of writer do you want to be?"
2. Have an explicit discussion about your roles. If your coaching relationship is relatively new, talk about the models you're basing your roles on: what experiences are shaping your role expectations? If your coaching

(continued)

relationship is ongoing, talk about how each of you think it has evolved. Was that evolution explicit or tacit?

3. To promote intellectual candour and reciprocal vulnerability, share a piece of painful reviewer feedback on a piece of writing that each person is trying to publish. Talk about how it makes each writer feel, and how they transform that into a productive way forward with the writing.

References

Aitchison, C. (2018). Writing an identity into being. In S. Carter & D. Laurs (Eds.), *Developing research writing: A handbook for supervisors and advisors* (pp. 193–197). London: Routledge.

Apramian, T., Cristancho, S., Watling, C., Ott, M., & Lingard, L. (2015). Thresholds of principle and preference: Exploring procedural variation in postgraduate surgical education. *Academic Medicine, 90*(11), S70–S76. https://doi.org/10.1097/ACM.0000000000000909.

Lamott, A. (1994). *Bird by bird: Some instructions on writing and life*. New York: Pantheon Books.

McGrath, L., Negretti, R., & Nicholls, K. (2019). Hidden expectations: Scaffolding subject specialists' genre knowledge of the assignments they set. *Higher Education, 78*, 835–853. https://doi.org/10.1007/s10734-019-00373-9.

Molloy, E., & Bearman, M. (2019). Embracing the tension between vulnerability and credibility: "Intellectual candour" in health professions education. *Medical Education, 53*(1), 32–41. https://doi.org/10.1111/medu.13649.

Vanstone, M. (2017). *Writing and the role of your supervisor*. http://www.meredithvanstone.com/assets/mv-grad_school_tips-writing_feedback.pdf. Accessed 28 Apr 2020.

Watling, C. J., & LaDonna, K. A. (2019). Where philosophy meets culture: Exploring how coaches conceptualise their roles. *Medical Education, 53*(5), 467–476. https://doi.org/10.1111/medu.13799.

Wellington, J. (2010). More than a matter of cognition: An exploration of affective writing problems of post-graduate students and their possible solutions. *Teaching in Higher Education, 15*(2), 135–150. https://doi.org/10.1080/13562511003619961.

Chapter 29
Cultivating a Writing Community

We regularly conduct master classes on writing research for publication. In these immersive, 3–4 day affairs, we walk participants through a range of conceptual, grammatical, and rhetorical strategies, and we give them plenty of time to write, with coaching on hand if they get stuck. For the most part, our goals are similar to those of this book: we hope to help them to think clearly about their research stories, and to get those stories on the page in compelling fashion.

But we have another goal. We aim to cultivate a writing *community*. We want participants to come together around the shared struggles and joys of writing. And – at least for a few days – we generally succeed. Participants listen intently as colleagues describe what they are trying to do in their writing. They offer each other polite endorsements at first, but quickly learn a language for supportive critique. "Your research is so interesting!" becomes "I love these ideas. Have you considered. . .?" and "I think you are burying a key point here. What if you tried it like this. . .?"

While we often manage to capture this magic in the retreat-like atmosphere of a writing course, we know that writing communities can be difficult to sustain in busy workplaces where writing competes with a thousand other priorities. In this chapter, we consider why and how we should make the time and space for writing communities in our professional worlds.

29.1 Why a Writing Community?

Learning

Writing communities are learning communities. They respond to an acknowledged need in the academic and clinical worlds that health researchers inhabit: researchers often feel that while the *products* of writing are valued in their settings, the *process*

L. Lingard, C. Watling, *Story, Not Study: 30 Brief Lessons to Inspire Health Researchers as Writers*, Innovation and Change in Professional Education 19, https://doi.org/10.1007/978-3-030-71363-8_29

of writing is unsupported (Murray et al. 2012). They need to learn to become better writers, but can easily spin their wheels. Writing communities offer traction and a path forward, functioning to "demystify the process of scholarly writing and publication" (Lee and Boud 2003, p. 190).

Learning occurs in the community's shared conversations around writing. Community members benefit from the feedback of other members. Ideally, these feedback conversations are supported by a shared language for talking about writing. In our own group, for example, we've made "problem/gap/hook" a verb, as in: "I've problem/gap/hooked a new paper I'm sketching out; would you mind taking a look and letting me know if I've been convincing?" For our group, this language signals that we're at a conceptualizing stage of the work, and that we are looking for feedback that targets that stage. Is the problem clear? Are you convinced there's a gap in how that problem is currently understood? And are you persuaded that filling that gap would matter?

Research on writing groups has suggested that, while members do indeed benefit from the feedback of other group members, they may gain even more from learning to be good critics (Aitchison 2009). As we've discussed in Chap. 26, the act of constructing feedback on others' writing is a tricky one. But it can be as transformative for the giver as for the receiver. Crafting a useful critique forces us to both name the problem and to experiment with possible solutions. It demands – and nurtures – a kind of storytelling facility that ultimately enhances the feedback giver's own work.

Identity

Communities shape identities. Most of us who write and publish research have other identities: we are clinicians or teachers or students or leaders or scientists, and it is these identities that tend to dominate. They direct how we describe ourselves to others, but also how we imagine ourselves. As a result, they may also shape how we value ourselves, how we prioritize our work tasks, and how we divide our time. If the writerly identity is always in the shadows, it can become challenging to give the act of writing our full attention.

The culture we inhabit often doesn't help. While academic faculty development has been described as a business of making and re-making identity (Lee and Boud 2003), the notion of developing an identity *as a writer* has been given little attention in universities and clinical settings (Murray 2012). Despite the pressure to publish endemic to these settings, the work of becoming a good writer often feels like it is valued less than other workplace activities – an unsettling paradox (Murray 2012). Writing can be viewed as self-serving, requiring an abdication of other, more pressing responsibilities. As a result, many academics think of writing as something to be done in their off hours (Murray 2012).

A writing community brings writing explicitly into "work hours", legitimizing it as a productive way to spend institutional time. It creates space and time where writing is paramount, requiring participants to focus on writing as a craft. Academic writers can sometimes be held back by anxiety that they aren't part of the writers' "club", and this anxiety and self-doubt can hold them back (Lee and Boud 2003). A writing community builds the writerly identity into their professional DNA, and with it the sense of confidence and belonging they require to succeed. But nurturing this writerly identity is political as well as personal. As researchers become comfortable granting their identities as writers equal status to their other professional identities, institutional acknowledgement and support may follow.

Motivation

A writing community often generates a sense of "mutual obligation" (Aitchison 2009, p. 906) that can be a draw for participants. Many academics report anxiety-provoking difficulties related to writing for publication, either due to the writing itself or to their challenges in balancing writing against competing activities. The "byproducts" of this anxiety are the writer's familiar foes: avoidance, procrastination, and lack of discipline (Murray et al. 2012). A community offers a line of defense: participants become responsible to their community, and exercising that responsibility means breaking through the distractions and making some progress.

One of us, for example, has a standing "Writing Wednesday" date with a colleague in another city. We set aside the same few hours most Wednesdays to write. We connect briefly beforehand, often by email, to share what we plan to work on; in doing so we articulate a specific commitment. Then we touch base briefly again afterward to share the products of our plan. Sometimes we trade drafts for feedback, but often we don't. Most times, what we are looking for is motivation rather than critique. We hold each other to account. Neither wants to disappoint the other by bailing on our plans, and that helps us both to maintain our writing momentum.

Of course, there's more to motivation than demands for accountability. We need to balance the sense of obligation we create with the spark of inspiration. A robust writing community can help to unearth joy in a craft that sometimes feels like a grind. A community offers a sense of audience that solitary writers often lack. Opportunities to connect with an audience – particularly an audience invested in each writer's success – can soothe the drudgery that writing can become. Remember that we aim, as writers, to join scholarly conversations, and conversations are social rather than solo acts.

29.2 Cultivating a Writing Community

Composition

Writing communities should be built with care. Competence, trust, and commitment are the foundations (Roulston et al. 2016). Competence means that community members have the skills to review and critique others' work. Content expertise matters less than the ability to contribute meaningfully to discussions about the writing process. Cross-disciplinary writing communities can thus be vibrant and productive. A lack of content familiarity may even free community members to focus on the writing itself – the quality of the arguments, the persuasiveness of the phrasing, the logic of the story. A diverse writing community may be the secret ingredient that enables us to write accessible stories that extend our scholarly reach.

Communities form for a multitude of reasons. Community members may share interests, challenges, or geography, or may simply be kindred spirits in their orientation to writing. Even if community members are at similar career stages, however, they will inevitably bring different levels of experience and writing skill to the table. The rule of engagement is reciprocity: regardless of experience or background, community members must be able to both take and give. In our master classes, we have been struck by the sense of community that can develop among individuals who vary in experience: a senior researcher with dozens of publications sometimes forms a productive relationship with a junior researcher working on their third paper, for example. Publishing experience doesn't always imply that a researcher feels in command of their writing, any more than a lack of published work implies that a researcher doesn't have confidence in their writing skills. Openness and humility likely matter more than experience, but community members need to feel capable of contributing to one another's progress. And communities do need to make room for less experienced members to join, acknowledging that the balance of taking to giving may shift as individuals learn, gain experience, and grow within the community.

Safety

A strong writing community supports risk-taking (Roulston et al. 2016). For this to be possible, trust and safety are non-negotiable. Creating spaces where writers can talk comfortably about their work is tricky, as such spaces can be fraught with issues of power, hierarchy, and autonomy (Lillis 2009). A strong writing community acknowledges this reality, while working to reduce the sense of vulnerability its members may experience. Sharing one's writing can be a personal and potentially threatening act. Participants in a community need to know that their communal work is confidential. The community needs to embrace a developmental focus for its shared work, and personal judgment must be absent from the critiques that are exchanged. Power and hierarchy need to move to the background, while collective purpose moves to the foreground (Lee and Boud 2003). Wenger's notion of a community of practice as a learning partnership is useful here (cited in Farnsworth et al. 2016), as partnerships imply a flattened hierarchy. A strong writing community builds trust by establishing clear goals and values around which the community can rally, and ground rules that the community commits to upholding. Each member should think about what is safe for them and trust their instincts. If you are in a writing group with someone you have a fraught relationship with (colleague, advisor, student) opening yourself up to feedback may be a threatening, and unproductive, experience.

Commitment

Even with competence and trust, communities fracture without commitment. A community of practice actually needs to be engaged in practice! Just as being a sports fan doesn't make you a better athlete, being a spectator in a writing community doesn't make you a better writer – and worse, it can drag the community down. First, writers in a community must be committed to their own writing tasks, and to the notion of iterative self-improvement. They need to be engaged in creating the raw materials that the community can take up. Second, they must be committed to the development of others within the community. Being a good citizen of a writing community means taking the task of critiquing others' work seriously. When a community embraces this principle – what some have called *mutuality* - community members will invest considerable energy in reviewing others' writing because they know their efforts will be returned when they offer up their own writing for review (Roulston et al. 2016). And as Lee and Boud (2003) eloquently note, commitment to others' development must reconcile writer autonomy and collective purpose:

> There is a delicate balance to be achieved between a productive taking-up of the agendas of particular members' projects by the group and an inappropriate appropriation of those agendas. At different points in the writing process, the group interactions might influence the shaping of a writing project, help to surface possibilities and directions, or take on a more editorial, readerly function. At all times, the groups' task was to assist a writer to position themself within their own writing, within the text and within the particular community of readers to whom the text was addressed. (p. 195)

We sometimes struggle to find this balance in our masterclasses. Writers may need to feel uncomfortable in order to stretch themselves as craftspeople, but their discomfort shouldn't grow out of a feeling that they have surrendered ownership of their work. When community input begins to reshape a writer's work, we need to pause and ask "Does this version remain true to your vision for your work?" Our most gratifying moments are when participants' own voices are amplified.

Are you keen to start a writing community? Figure 29.1 offers a set of ground rules that can help to guide you:

29.3 Conclusion

Writing may often be solitary, but it needn't be lonely. The support and solidarity of a community can be emotionally sustaining for writers. But a strong writing community does more than offer moral support. It can be the lightning-in-a-bottle necessary to jump start stalled writing, stimulate learning, and accelerate progress. And if we're lucky, a writing community may amplify the joy and satisfaction that the craft offers.

- Establish the community as a safe and confidential space to work on writing. What happens in the community stays in the community.
- Require a commitment as the price of membership in the community. Members need to commit to working on (and sharing) their own writing, *and* to constructively critiquing their colleagues' writing.
- Develop a shared language for talking about writing. (Tip: this book can help!)
- Encourage diversity in the community; a shared interest in writing matters more than shared research or disciplinary expertise.
- Create a schedule of community activities, and encourage members to put them in their work calendars.
- Encourage experimentation. Push each other to stretch as writers.
- For more seasoned writers: share your writing struggles with more junior members of the community. They'll find it immensely reassuring.
- For less experienced writers: simply share your perspective as a reader. Your authentic reactions to others' writing will be enlightening for them.
- Celebrate writing and publishing successes, but also create space for productively debriefing failures as a community.

Fig. 29.1   Ground rules for a successful writing community

See One, Do One, Teach One

1. Sow the seeds of a writing community by inviting a small group of colleagues to join you. As you contemplate who to invite, consider:

   (a) Experience
   (b) Diversity of perspectives
   (c) Shared commitment

2. With your community members invited, brainstorm to settle on shared goals for the community. Consider what community members need: motivation? critical feedback? accountability? Use Fig. 29.1 as a guide for the conversation, if helpful.

3. Design a few activities that level the playing field in communities with writers of varied experience. For example, invite experienced writers to share their worst reviews, and to discuss how they handled them and (hopefully!) rebounded. Or invite more novice writers to share the best tip about writing they have received, and to offer an example of their efforts to incorporate that tip into their work.

References

Aitchison, C. (2009). Writing groups for doctoral education. *Studies in Higher Education, 4*(8), 905–916. https://doi.org/10.1080/03075070902785580.

Farnsworth, V., Kleanthous, I., & Wenger-Trayner, E. (2016). Communities of practice as a social theory of learning: A conversation with Etienne Wenger. *British Journal of Educational Studies, 64*(2), 139–160. https://doi.org/10.1080/00071005.2015.1133799.

Lee, A., & Boud, D. (2003). Writing groups, change and academic identity: Research development as local practice. *Studies in Higher Education, 28*(2), 187–200. https://doi.org/10.1080/0307507032000058109.

Lillis, T. (2009). Bringing writers' voices to writing research: Talk around research. In S. Parker, A. Carter, & T. Lillis (Eds.), *Why writing matters: Issues of identity in writing research and pedagogy* (Vol. 12, pp. 169–188). Amsterdam: John Benjamins Publishing.

Murray, R. (2012). Developing a community of research practice. *British Educational Research Journal, 38*(5), 783–800. https://doi.org/10.1080/01411926.2011.583635.

Murray, R., Steckley, L., & MacLeod, I. (2012). Research leadership in writing for publication: A theoretical framework. *British Educational Research Journal, 38*(5), 765–778. https://doi.org/10.1080/01411926.2011.580049.

Roulston, K., Teitelbaum, D., Chang, B., & Butchart, R. (2016). Strategies for developing a writing community for doctoral students. *International Journal for Researcher Development, 7*(2), 198–210. https://doi.org/10.1108/IJRD-02-2016-0003.

Chapter 30
Successfully Navigating the Peer Review Process

Submitting your completed manuscript is a huge achievement. But submitted is not published. Between the pinnacles of submission and publication lies the valley of peer review. Here, reviewers critique your work, editors translate those critiques into recommendations, and you use those recommendations to produce a strengthened manuscript that will, hopefully, be accepted for publication. Any writer who has traversed this valley knows it can be dark and difficult terrain. We've all had the experience of stumbling, and of turning back to start the journey all over again. This chapter offers strategies to navigate the peer review process successfully by understanding the journal review system, decoding reviewer comments, and crafting effective responses.

30.1 Understanding the System

There are a number of decision points along the route from submission to acceptance. First, your submission is reviewed by the editor or a journal staff member to judge its general relevance, quality, and originality. If deemed unacceptable at this stage, it will be "desk rejected". Desk rejections take the form of a generic email thanking you for your submission and informing you that the journal is not interested. They often signal that the journal is not having this conversation. If this initial review is positive, however, your manuscript will be assigned to an associate (or 'handling') editor who is tasked with finding peer reviewers.

Peer review is voluntary, unpaid work by busy academics and clinicians whose institutions may not meaningfully recognize it as a scholarly contribution. Therefore, it is increasingly difficult to find reviewers (Tite and Schroter 2007), and associate editors must cast an ever-widening net to find reviewers for the manuscripts they oversee. Because of this, reviewers may have less methodological or content expertise than you might have hoped for, thus the need to prepare your work for judgment

L. Lingard, C. Watling, *Story, Not Study: 30 Brief Lessons to Inspire Health Researchers as Writers*, Innovation and Change in Professional Education 19, https://doi.org/10.1007/978-3-030-71363-8_30

by educated and interested non-experts. Reviews are guided by a set of criteria dictated by the journal, such as the originality of the work, rigor of the methodological procedures, and clarity of the writing. Reviews are usually blinded, meaning the reviewers do not know who the authors are, and anonymous, meaning you don't know who your reviewers are. They are intended to be constructive, but many writers experience them otherwise. A recent analysis of reviews from 10 randomly selected BioMed Central (BMC) journals described three reviewer types – nurturing, begrudged and blasé – and found that a number of factors beyond manuscript quality influenced the nature of reviews (Le Sueur et al. 2020). Hyland and Jiang's (2020) "anatomy" of harsh peer reviews from shitmyreviewerssay.tumblr.com identified the linguistic features that set these texts apart from expectations of collegial behaviour; their results suggest both why such reviews are so wounding and how reviewers might avoid inflicting such injuries on their colleagues. Some journals have introduced an option for reviewers to choose to sign their reviews, in an effort to promote professionalism and transparency in the process.

Once reviews have been conducted, the associate editor should summarize key issues and give you guidance regarding how to reconcile conflicting opinions. Sometimes editors add their own critiques, as in this review one of us recently received:

> Your manuscript was well-received by our reviewers and I can certainly appreciate why they think it has such value. I do, however, have a few more substantial concerns than those reported below that I will need to see addressed before a final decision can be made.

Associate editors have a pivotal role, and you shouldn't underestimate their authority. While the decision email from the journal is usually signed by the Editor, the associate editor is often the primary audience for your efforts to revise and resubmit. You should take very seriously any guidance or additional criticism they offer.

If your manuscript undergoes peer review, you will receive one of three possible decisions: Accept, Revise and Resubmit (minor or major revisions), or Reject. The first is vanishingly rare in health services research; in our combined 40+ years of experience, only three times have we experienced an acceptance with no revisions. The second possibility is that you will be asked to revise and resubmit. In this case, you will be given a timeframe (usually 1–3 months) for the resubmission. Many journals distinguish between major and minor revisions, but don't get hung up on these labels. We have found that revisions labelled "major' can sometimes look pretty innocuous, while those labelled 'minor' can sometimes require heavy lifting. Certainly don't read 'Major Revision' to mean that the journal doesn't want your manuscript. Major or minor, a revise and resubmit decision is a foot in the door!

The third possibility is a Reject decision. Rejection is painful, no matter how many papers you've published. However, it still offers an opportunity to improve your paper and you should consider the reviewer comments even though you are not resubmitting to this particular journal. Health research domains are a relatively small worlds and many journals draw on the same reviewer pool, so you could very well encounter that reviewer again. If you can improve your manuscript based on their feedback, it will help your next submission. Furthermore, some journals now offer the opportunity to include any previous reviews and your responses to them when you submit a manuscript that has been previously rejected. This approach is growing in popularity, as it avoids wasting reviewer effort and may allow a journal to make a decision without requiring a complete set of additional reviews (Ellaway et al. 2020).

30.2 Decoding the Reviews

Engaging with your reviews is not always an easy task. As Thomson and Kamler (2013) note, journal reviews are 'coded' and the codes vary across discourse communities and disciplines. Consequently, understanding what reviewers want from you can require considerable reading between the lines. Consider this reviewer comment:

> Perhaps it might be helpful to explore the conceptual and theoretical issues around gender and reflect on how these fundamentally shape the way power works in clinical interactions in much more depth.

You might understandably perceive some contradictions in this comment. The modality of "perhaps" and "might be helpful" could be read as a suggestion, while phrases like "fundamentally" and "in much more depth" signal a request for substantial rethinking of key ideas. A seasoned writer will probably recognize the modality as a politeness strategy, interpret the request to "explore the conceptual and theoretical issues" as a strong criticism that the paper is conceptually weak, and understand "reflect on" in this context to mean "seriously rework" rather than "think a bit about". But a writer with less experience might not be sure whether this reviewer is saying "you must" or "you could consider".

Getting this right is critical: one of the main reasons that revised and resubmitted manuscripts get rejected is a failure to engage meaningfully with the critique. We tend to like what we've written, so we lean towards interpreting 'minor revisions' as light tinkering and 'major revisions' as minor revisions. Therefore, it is important to decode your reviews carefully. Comments usually fall into a finite set of general themes:

- Gaps in the literature review setting up the work
- Points of clarification or elaboration of the theoretical framing
- Requests for details of or disputes with methodological procedures
- Issues with the nature, display, or interpretation of the results
- Problems with the coherence of the story
- Attention to the 'so what' of the work
- Queries about the originality of the contribution
- Concerns about the scope of the conclusions
- Technical flags (length, formatting, English, ethical approvals)

Table 30.1 Decoding reviewer comments

Theme	Reviewer comment	Decoded meaning(s)	Next steps
Gaps in the literature review setting up the work	"There is much relevant research on professionalism issues during clerkship and the authors would do well to cite it."	You excluded sources that this reviewer finds essential.	Ascertain what these are and decide whether/how to integrate them.
		You may have overlooked THIS reviewer's work.	Check what they've published.
		You have treated as common knowledge aspects of this problem that need to be evidenced.	Check your introduction for common sense statements that need conversion to knowledge claims.
	"The background is long and detailed with over 25 references, but it doesn't give a strong sense of why this study is necessary."	Your review is thorough but the gap your work fills is not clear enough.	Create an argument for what's missing, not just a listing of what's known.
		Your review is meandering, including material that is distracting the reader from the line of argument.	Select and organize the knowledge claims carefully: Remove those that don't contribute to the logic.
	"The review of CBME and programmatic assessment literatures is sound, but other issues (e.g., failure to fail) are also relevant and need attention here."	There are relevant domains missing in your literature review.	Add these paragraphs to thoroughly contextualize the work.
		The reviewer is interested in these other domains and wonders if you have considered their relevance.	Demonstrate that you are aware of these issues but deflect (with references) the expectation that they are central here.

Within these themes, however, comments vary a great deal in how they are worded. This affects how you decode them and, therefore, how you will respond. Table 30.1 offers sample comments around the theme of gaps in the literature review, suggests some decoded meanings, and illustrates how the decoding influences possible next steps.

As these examples demonstrate, reviewer comments can be decoded in multiple ways. Experience can help you to judge, for instance, that in the last example you may not need to include the literature on failure to fail; instead, you could signal that you are aware of it and deflect the expectation that it's central to your argument.

Another factor in how we decode reviewer comments is the emotional response they provoke in us. Feedback on our writing feels personal. We can feel anger or shame when reviewers tell us our work has not met the bar. These feelings produce various responses. Some writers don't even open the emailed decision from the journal for a few days, as they muster the courage to read it. Some look at the decision immediately and scan the comments, but don't take it all in until a subsequent read. Some writers come out swinging after reading critiques of their work; hopefully, they process this response over coffee with a colleague rather than on email with the journal! Some die a little inside, quietly tucking the manuscript into a drawer to gather dust and pledging never to tell a soul.

Our first decoding of reviewer comments is likely skewed by our emotions. For that reason, we recommend the 48-hour rule: take 2 days to lick your wounds and process the emotions. But only 48 hours! Don't let a reviewed manuscript languish; anything other than a Reject decision should be approached as an opportunity. The other strategy for getting past that first emotional response – and ensuring it doesn't unduly color the reading of the reviews – is to engage what Thomson and Kamler (2013) refer to as a "publication broker" (p. 134) to help you systematically analyze them. This can be an experienced co-author, but there is value in sharing your reviews with someone outside the writing team who can bring both experience and objectivity to the table. This individual can help novice writers to process the threat to their budding identities as writers -- and more seasoned writers to calm the surge of imposter syndrome – provoked by a negative set of reviews.

Particularly difficult to process are nasty reviews. Peer review should be a collegial, respectful enterprise, but the popular Reviewer 2 meme in social media suggests that many writers experience it otherwise ("Shit My Reviewers Say" n.d.). It's not that your *particular* Reviewer 2 is more likely to give you a nasty review than reviewers 1 or 3 (Peterson 2020). Rather, Reviewer 2 is a symbol of the peer reviewer who is aggressive, rude, vague, smug, self-absorbed, committed to pet issues, theories and methodologies, and unwilling to give the benefit of the doubt or view the authors as peers. Linguistically, these reviews abound with features such as attitude markers (e.g., verbs like "reject", sentence adverbs like "absurdly", and adjectives like "illogical"), self-mention (e.g., "I cannot possibly imagine"), and boosters (e.g., "the manuscript is utterly ridiculous") (Hyland and Jiang 2020). Reviews exemplifying such characteristics are hard for anyone to take; however, they may disproportionately harm underrepresented groups (Silbiger and Stubler 2019). Efforts to improve the quality and tone of reviews include "open peer review", in which reviewers can opt (or are required, depending on the journal) to sign their reviews. Beyond signing, other features of open review may also promote better review quality and tone. For example, some journals now share with all reviewers both the editor's decision and the full set of reviews. This makes reviewers more publicly accountable for their remarks and allows them the opportunity to read other reviewers' comments. We have found that this is an educational experience because we see that other reviewers respond differently than we do, they note other problems and strengths, and, sometimes, they teach us turns of phrase that we go on to use to make difficult feedback more digestible.

30.3 Crafting Your Response

Writers send two documents back to the journal when they revise and resubmit: the revised manuscript and a response to reviews letter. We consider each of these in turn.

The Revised Manuscript

You've carefully read through the many pages of reviews. You've found a "publication broker" to help you decode them. Now you need a revision plan that prioritizes and organizes them. Start by analyzing all the materials (including editor and associate editor email text) for "action points" (Silvia 2019). Reviews can be meandering and conversational, so it helps to distinguish reflections from requirements. Highlighting action points focuses your attention on what the journal wants you to do differently.

When writers revise and resubmit, they don't slavishly obey every request for changes to the manuscript. Some requests are asking for a different study or paper altogether, like when the reviewer suggests that your multiple case study would have been better as a critical narrative inquiry. Or they wish your survey sample had included family caregivers, not just patients. Therefore, it helps to have a system for sorting requests. Try listing all the action points you identified and asking yourself the following questions about each one:

- Is this a request for more, for less, or for something altogether different?
- Does it require a major rethink or a minor rewrite?
- Do I want to incorporate this suggestion, or not?
- If not, what is my rationale for not making the change?

Using these questions to analyze the action points in your reviews should give you a sense of whether you're achieving some balance between integrating suggestions and holding your ground. There is no perfect equation for this, but, generally speaking, you should aim to incorporate all the suggestions that you can, and be selective and strategic about those that you refuse. Researchers often find themselves with more methodological expertise than their reviewers, and therefore they may need to decline certain suggestions in order to maintain credibility within the larger research community. In such cases, a thoughtful response is required rather than a revision. The keyword here is 'thoughtful'. If your response to reviews letter reads as a litany of "yeah, buts" in which you dismiss reviewer's suggestions, you will come across as not engaging meaningfully with the review process. And you might find yourself in receipt of an email like this one, which we received some years ago and have taken to heart:

> This is a slightly revised version of a paper reporting results of a study of XXX. I am disappointed by the revisions offered by the authors. They have indirectly and insufficiently addressed my concerns and they have deflected several of the suggestions of the reviewers.

Once you have a plan and revisions are well underway, don't forget to consider how the changes will impact the overall coherence of the manuscript. Beware the butterfly effect: an edit on page 1 can unexpectedly affect the argument on page 7. Transitions will need attention after reworking sentences, paragraphs and sections. Efforts to shorten the text, such as tightening up the background, will mean that later sections that assumed now-deleted material will need refining. Elaborations of the Discussion should prompt a rethink of the Introduction so that the storyline hangs

Reviewer comment	Description of revisions	Location of revisions
Reviewer 1		
…		
…		
Reviewer 2		
…		

Fig. 30.1 A response to reviews template

together. And the Abstract will undoubtedly need attention to accurately reflect the revision.

The Response to Reviews Letter

Almost as important as your revised manuscript is the letter you write explaining your revision. We all write 'response to review' letters but we rarely see anyone else's. They are "occluded texts" (Swales 1990): commonplace, backstage genres that we tend to treat as administrative rather than academic. Don't be fooled: they can make or break your resubmission. Content, organization, and tone are all critical.

In terms of content, the letter should contain summary, description, and argumentation. It summarizes the action points in the peer review. It describes what you've changed in the manuscript and where those changes can be found. And it argues on one of three fronts: how the changes satisfy the review comments, why you're offering something other than what was requested, or why you are not accommodating a reviewer request.

In terms of organization, there are two general approaches: a table or a narrative. In either format, your goal is to make it as easy as possible for the overworked editor to clearly see what you've done. Some journals require a tabular response that presents each reviewer comment separately, as in the following adapted example (Fig. 30.1) (AM Rounds 2019).

Such a table is a great way of organizing your response as you go through the reviews, ensuring you've adequately dealt with all issues. However, the tabular format has two main drawbacks. It can produce a letter that is many pages long and repetitive, particularly when reviewers comment on similar issues in the paper. You can address this by organizing the table by manuscript sections (Introduction, Methods, Results, Discussion) and listing reviewer and editor points within them. However, this solution doesn't address another problem of the tabular format, which is its inability to clearly distinguish between substantive action points and minor technical issues. You don't want the tabular format to detract from your ability to create a coherent and convincing argument in your response letter. A hybrid letter can be a good compromise, as long as you to clearly orient the reader in the opening, as the following example does:

Thank you for opportunity to revise and resubmit our manuscript. We have carefully considered the editor and reviewer comments, which have helped us to strengthen our presentation of our research. Some substantial issues were flagged by multiple reviewers. For coherence, we have gathered these into three main paragraphs at the beginning of this response letter, followed by a tabular listing of all the remaining comments and our responses, organized by IMRD structure.

The following extract exemplifies a paragraph that collects all the comments related to a substantive issue. And it illustrates how <u>summary</u>, *description* and **argumentation** can be woven together. The letter doesn't simply say "thank you for this important comment" and "here is what we've done in response" or "you've missed the point". It uses argumentation to interpret the comment, place it in a larger context (here, the requirements of this methodology) and educate when necessary:

> <u>Two of the reviewers and the associate editor requested more information about the interviews, including "the number of possible participants", "the extent to which participants were representative of the population", the "content of the interview protocol", and "more attention to the relationship between the participants and the researchers".</u> *We have included additional contextual information at the start of the Methods section (p2), including the total number of residents at the institution where most of the work took place and the range of disciplines in which residents there train.* **Because the goal of sampling in our method-ology is not to produce generalizations about the population but rather to describe complex social experiences in depth[3], it is not appropriate for us to make claims about representing the population. However, the provision of this information should help readers judge the extent to which our sample of 20 residents reflects the diversity of this group, which we understand to be the spirit of this reviewer question.** *The original interview protocol is now included (Appendix 3),* and ***on page 3 we explain the main alterations to this protocol that occurred during theoretical sampling.*** *We have clarified on page 3 that the interviews were conducted by a research assistant with no relationship to the participants.*

Notice the sentence that is both bolded and italicized: "on page 3 we explain the main alterations to this protocol that occurred during theoretical sampling". This both describes the change and, at the same time, does some educating. To ensure that readers less familiar with the methodology don't incorrectly assume that the inter-view protocol was static throughout the course of the data collection, the authors explain the main alterations that were made to it. This was not requested by the reviewer, but it is a necessary elaboration so that fulfilling their request does not create confusion.

The tone of the letter is also key. You don't need to be overly diffident, but neither should you be defensive or arrogant. Your letter is a respectful argument, particularly when you are not straightforwardly implementing a reviewer's suggestion. Write the letter as though the reviewers will read it. Because they just might. Particularly when revisions are major, the manuscript may go back to the same reviewers for their judgment on how convincingly it has satisfied the requests for revision. Finally, just as you would have your co-authors review the revised manuscript, have them review the response letter. They will be able to point out where the tone might be problem-atic, so that you can refine it prior to submitting.

30.4 Conclusion

Any invitation to revise and resubmit your manuscript is an opportunity that puts you one step closer to publication. Don't stumble in these last steps of the journey. Knowing how the journal review system works will help you to decode reviewer comments accurately, maximizing the likelihood that your revised manuscript will satisfy. And attending to the content, structure, and tone of your response letter will ensure that you engage effectively in this conversation with journal representatives.

See One, Do One, Teach One
1. Pull out your most recent set of reviews and categorize the reviewer comments under "revise as requested", "revise with caveats", or "hold my ground". Take note of the balance of the items in each category.
2. Craft a rationale for each of the "hold my ground" items that is a) grounded in science, and b) passes the "tone test" with an experienced colleague from outside the research team.
3. Identify the single most irritating reviewer comment. Write the response that comes from your gut, save it in a file, and read it again in a week. With the benefit of a little time, what do you notice about your tone? Has your attitude toward the comment changed? What revising do you need to do before it is fit to send?

References

AM Rounds: Beyond the pages of Academic Medicine. (2019, September 13). *Addressing reviewer comments recap: Key takeaways and additional resources*. http://academicmedicineblog.org/addressing-reviewer-comments-recap-key-takeaways-and-additional-resources/. Accessed 9 Sept 2020.

Ellaway, R., Tolsgaard, M., & Norman, G. (2020). Peer review is not a lottery: AHSE's fast track. *Advances in Health Science Education, 25*, 519–521. https://doi.org/10.1007/s10459-020-09981-y.

Hyland, K., & Jiang, F. K. (2020). "This work is antithetical to the spirit of research": An anatomy of harsh peer reviews. *Journal of English for Academic Purposes, 46*, 100867.

Le Sueur, H., Dagliati, A., Buchan, I., Whetton, A. D., Martin, G. P., Dornan, T., et al. (2020). Pride and prejudice – What can we learn from peer review? *Medical Teacher, 42*(9), 1012–1018. https://doi.org/10.1080/0142159X.2020.1774527.

Peterson, D. A. M. (2020). Dear reviewer 2: Go F' yourself. *Social Science Quarterly, 101*(4), 1648–1652. https://doi.org/10.1111/ssqu.12824.

Shit my reviewers say. (n.d.). *Tumblr*. https://shitmyreviewerssay.tumblr.com/. Accessed 4 Sept 2020.

Silbiger, N. J., & Stubler, A. D. (2019). Unprofessional peer reviews disproportionately harm underrepresented groups in STEM. *Peer Journal: Life & Environment, 7*, e8247. https://doi.org/10.7717/peerj.8247.

Silvia, P. J. (2019). *How to write a lot: A guide to productive academic writing* (2nd ed.). Washington, DC: American Psychological Association.

Swales, J. (1990). *Genre analysis: English in academic and research settings*. Cambridge: Cambridge University Press.

Thomson, P., & Kamler, B. (2013). *Writing for peer-reviewed journals: Strategies for getting published*. London: Routledge.

Tite, L., & Schroter, S. (2007). Why do peer reviewers decline to review? A survey. *Journal of Epidemiology and Community Health, 61*(1), 9–12. https://doi.org/10.1136/jech.2006.049817.

Correction to: Get Control of Your Commas

Correction to:
Chapter 14 in: L. Lingard, C. Watling, *Story, Not Study:*
***30 Brief Lessons to Inspire Health Researchers as Writers*,**
Innovation and Change in Professional Education 19,
https://doi.org/10.1007/978-3-030-71363-8_14

The book was inadvertently published with typographical error in epigraph. The text has now been corrected in the chapter.

The updated version of the chapter can be found at
https://doi.org/10.1007/978-3-030-71363-8_14

L. Lingard, C. Watling, *Story, Not Study: 30 Brief Lessons to Inspire Health
Researchers as Writers*, Innovation and Change in Professional Education 19,
https://doi.org/10.1007/978-3-030-71363-8_31

Epilogue

Bringing our Conversation to a Close

We suspect that very few of you will have read these chapters in order, from beginning to end. Rather, we anticipate that, as busy health researchers, you will have dipped in and out of this book opportunistically. We hope you found helpful strategies for honing the story in your manuscript, clear explanations for diagnosing and improving grammar challenges, and inspiration for providing feedback and support to other writers. We hope you dog-eared pages and highlighted passages. We hope you photocopied the Tables you found most helpful and taped them to the wall in your writing area. We hope you pirated the See One, Do One, Teach One exercises for use with your students. We hope you purchased some of the books in the references for your bedtime reading pile. Finally, we hope you perceive yourself *as a writer*, one who is committed to using their study to tell a story that matters in the world.

Thank you for engaging with us in this conversation about the craft of scientific writing. We had so much fun, we may need to do this again!

Index

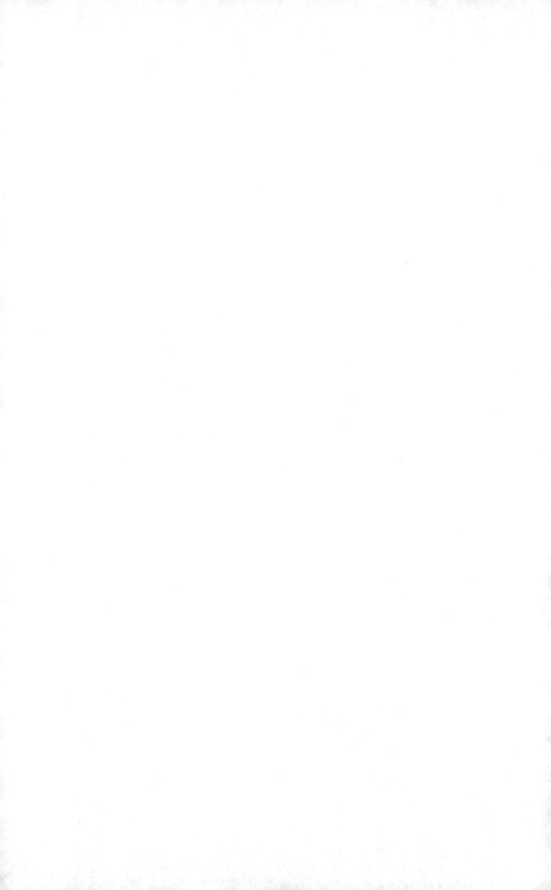

CPSIA information can be obtained
at www.ICGtesting.com
Printed in the USA
BVHW031117230622
640497BV00008B/593

9 783030 713652